Through Northern Eyes

Through Northern Eyes

by

James Graham Gillan, M.D., F.R.C.S.(C)
Ophthalmologist

University of Calgary Press

0224444

© 1991 James Graham Gillan. All rights reserved

University of Calgary Press
2500 University Drive N.W.
Calgary, Alberta, Canada T2N 1N4

Canadian Cataloguing in Publication Data

Gillan, James Graham, 1915–
   Through northern eyes

Includes index.
ISBN 1-895176-00-X (soft cover)
ISBN 1-895176-16-6 (hard cover)

   1. Gillan, James Graham. 2. Ophthalmologists—
Canada, Northern—Biography. 3. Ophthalmology—
Canada, Northern—History. I. Title.

RE36.G5A3 1991   617.7′092   C91-091759-0

Cover design by Rhae Ann Bromley

Printed in Canada by Friesen Printers

∞ This book is printed on acid-free paper.

15 JUL 1992

To my wife Annelise

who shares my life and my adventures

Contents

Foreword

IN TIMES WHEN young physicians are anxious to move into busy practice, there seems less inclination to travel or to learn more about the greater world. Urbanization is one price paid for education. This is a pity, for the Canadian Northlands are fascinating places.

I first came across Graham Gillan's name when I visited Labrador in 1969. Of Scottish origin and the son of missionary parents, he had for several years made time from a busy ophthalmic practice in Toronto to pursue his interest in the care of people in remote locations. He had served with the Grenfell Association, as it was at that time, visiting both Newfoundland and Labrador over many years. Later, as retirement approached, he changed his location to the Northwest Territories, where he supervised eye care in that vast region while living in Yellowknife.

Wherever he travelled, he had the knack of asking those simple questions which open research opportunities. Sometimes the questions concerned hereditary eye diseases, sometimes an unusual prevalence of some particular disorder. He would then contact a colleague in a university centre, and often a paper would result.

The combination of curiosity about eye diseases, his concern for work in the North, and his love of people, led him to reflect on perspectives in medicine, and on problems of remote area care. It was therefore no surprise when following retirement he took to writing. It is a privilege to contribute this foreword for an unusual friend.

Henry Wyatt, Chairman
Department of Ophthalmology
University of Alberta

Preface

---

*T*HROUGH NORTHERN EYES is a rare first-person account by a northern medical practitioner. While several generations of southern professionals have gone North to work, very few have managed to record their experiences for the benefit of current northern residents and new generations of indigenous and incoming professionals. As a result the history of northern development and health care delivery is left by default to the grey literature of unpublished letters, memoirs and photographs, and the professional historian who builds published reality from private sources. Dr. Gillan has made an important contribution to first-person "I was there" Canadian history in this book.

He also reveals through his writing a great deal about himself and his motivation to work in what southerners often think of as remote hinterland communities. As the child of missionary parents and a strongly motivated Christian he took his faith North. However, he was not quick to judge others and in the book the reader witnesses the evolution of a practical, well-prepared and generous northerner. He drove the long white ice roads at 40 degrees below, he risked his life in bush aircraft, he served his patients before nine and after five and he kept his sense of humour in the face of remote decisions taken in Ottawa that affected his life in Frobisher Bay.

A standard northerner's criticism of recent northern literature goes as follows: if the southern journalist comes North for a day he becomes an expert and writes a feature article; if he stays for a month he publishes the definitive book; but if he stays for a year he loses the ability to write at all, being simply overwhelmed by the beauty, change and complexity of the North. Well thank God for Dr. Gillan; he stayed more than a year and he wrote the book!

One must also thank Canadian publishers who share Dr. Gillan's dream of telling the story of northern development at first hand. In their absence we are destined to form images of our northern heritage based on Hollywood, novels, academic history and hearsay. With the advent of VHS and the satellite dish it is just as easy to watch "North to Alaska" in Fort Good Hope as it is in Calgary. On both sides of the Arctic Circle children are now being socialized by electronic media and living rooms are places where people watch the flickering images of television in rapt silence. Dr. Gillan's North was a different place and his living room was a vibrant, vocal, cross-cultural feast. By reading this book you can re-enter that room and learn first-hand about northern development through Dr. Gillan's eyes.

Mike Robinson
Executive Director and Adjunct Professor
Arctic Institute of North America

Acknowledgements

EVERY BOOK IS like a vehicle produced by many workers, where the author acts only as spark plug and battery to make it go. Even unknowingly, many people and incidents play a part. Long-ago, as well as recent, influences contribute: my parents, who thought and taught that other people were important and my medical instructors who held the old standards of patient priority.

Obviously, I cannot acknowledge all the people who entered into the making of this work. However, I tender thanks to some of the recent contributors: Miss U. J. Hull, S.R.N., for pictures of Newfoundland and Labrador; Mr. Michael Robinson of the Arctic Institute of North America for his kind Preface and helpfulness in providing sources of information; Mr. Terry Garvin for information on early conditions at Rae-Edzo; Dr. Don Smith, Department of History, The University of Calgary, for tracing the rare document, "The Story of a National Crime," and for giving helpful advice as well; Dr. Henry Wyatt for his generous Foreword; Drs. Gordon Johnson and W. G. Pearce for helpful comments; Dr. James Watt for illustrations; the Medical Library Researchers for their courtesy and help; Mr. John Parker for information on Elizabeth Cass; Mr. Peter Schledermann of the Arctic Institute for his advice; Rod Chapman for copyediting; Bill Matheson for preparing the maps; Christopher Blackburn for the index, and finally, Linda Cameron and her staff at the University of Calgary Press for their extensive help and patience.

For permission to reproduce excerpts from already published manuscripts, I would like to acknowledge McGraw-Hill Ryerson Limited, for the quote from F. W. Rowe's *The Development of Education in Newfoundland* (Toronto: Ryerson Press, 1964), and Joseph R. Smallwood, for the quotes from his book, *I Chose Canada* (Toronto: Macmillan, 1973).

1 / *What am I doing here?*

Fear not that life may come to an end, but that it never has had
a beginning.

John Henry Newman

THE PILOT LOWERED the flaps, pushed the joystick and
descended until the skis hit the snow-covered runway. Only
some oil drums, one marked with a flag, indicated this was a
Labrador airstrip.

It was February 1964, and I was sitting beside the pilot of a
de Havilland Otter M.I.T. ("Mike Indian Tango," as they called
her on the radio) Grenfell Mission air ambulance. "We're
supposed to meet a patient from Black Tickle[1] here," the pilot
said. "We'll wait a few minutes to see if he shows."

There was no house in sight. In the air ambulance were five
patients being transferred from small fishing outposts to hospital at St. Anthony, Newfoundland, and two nurses. The pilot
pointed to a spot on the hill over which two figures could be
seen pulling a qamutiik, an Inuit sleigh usually harnessed to
dogs or to a snowmobile. Two sons were dragging their sick
father from the nearby village of Black Tickle. They soon put
him aboard and the plane quickly accelerated down the snow-
covered runway. When we were airborne, we turned towards
Port Hope Simpson, another outpost community.

"What am I doing here?" I asked myself as we flew south.
In 1963, I had received a letter from a young physician colleague who had recently left Toronto to work with the Grenfell
Mission. The letter informed me that Dr. Eleanor Faye, who had
been visiting St. Anthony for one month each year from New
York, would not be available for further visits and the coast
would have no ophthalmologist. Could I come and help?

This was followed only a few days later by a letter from Dr. Gordon Thomas,[2] medical superintendent of the Grenfell Mission. This stated that he had been given my name, and that he was glad I was prepared to help. Both of these doctors appeared to be more sure of me than I was of myself!

The challenge had been issued. Could I, should I, and would I accept it?

Could I? I was busy. I had come to Toronto about fifteen years before after five years with the British Armed Forces, and some service with the Eye Hospital of St. John of Jerusalem.[3] After the evacuation of the British women and children, I resigned my post in Jerusalem and followed my Canadian wife to Canada. While I had obtained my general medical degree from Glasgow University in 1939, and a British specialist degree in ophthalmology from the College of Physicians and Surgeons of London, I had to obtain equivalent degrees in Canada. Having prepared myself in this way, I had obtained appointments at three of the hospitals on the periphery of Metropolitan Toronto. I looked at my schedule. As it was, I had too little time for family, holidays and conferences.

Should I? I suppose I always knew what I should do, but I was afraid. Something about this knock on the door told me that if I opened it even a little, I would never be quite the same. Now I was nearly fifty. I had been trying to do something for missionary work, as I taught treatment of eye disease at the Missionary Health Institute, where training was given to young people devoting their lives to the service of others. Also I belonged to the Evangelical Missionary Aid Society, and the Christian Medical Society. Short-term service is usual for members of both these groups. There seemed to be no doubt as to what I should do. But again the warning voice said: "You will not be able to stop at one trip—are you prepared to go all the way?"

Would I go? It was a test of my moral fibre. A domestic matter gave me a temporary excuse, so I wrote that I would not be able to visit St. Anthony at that time. But it is easier to make such a decision than to live with it. Christmas is a time for giving. That Christmas I could no longer be content with giving

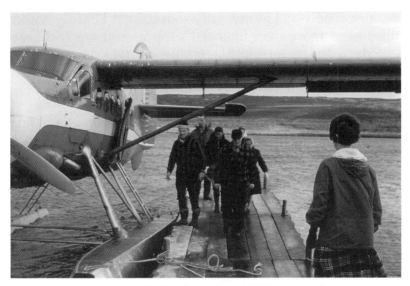

De Havilland Otter M.I.T.

presents—I realized I had to give myself more fully to the service of others.

Meanwhile, even as the pressure of greater involvement in Newfoundland was increasing for me, things had been changing in Toronto. I had come to Canada when Toronto was exploding with municipalities—each with their own ideas of need and priorities. Some municipalities wanted hospitals and had budgeted for them. York Township, for example, arranged to build the Northwestern General Hospital on Keele Street. The idea was that specialists who wanted staff privileges should have practices within the township and be ratepayers. Similarly, the Seventh-Day Adventist church was anxious to build a hospital in North York, which became the North York Branson Hospital.

For a time I was alone as an ophthalmologist in each of these hospitals, and I also did considerable surgery in a small private hospital called Bethesda run by the Missionary Health Institute. I even became chairman of this group, which was hoping to become a general hospital in Willowdale. As I lived in Etobicoke, I was in the founding group for Queensway Hospital, and after it was completed I also had privileges there.

So absorbed was I in my daily rounds that I hardly realized families need more than financial support and we had grown apart. My wife left for Florida, taking my two daughters who were enrolled in high school and university. While my wife did find work, the expense of a second home and periodic visits still added to my load.

I did ask a senior member of the Florida medical establishment about my chances of practising in Florida. He told me there was an unwritten policy to withhold hospital appointments from doctors of my age who had already practised in the north. The hospitals disliked "snow birds," who practised in the winter in the south but returned north during the summer months when the full-time resident ophthalmologists were anxious to go on vacation. This left emergency departments too exposed. Florida was interested in young Canadian doctors only if they would become permanent residents.

For me it was too risky economically, especially since it was uncertain I would be able to repair the rift in family relationships. Continuing my practice, with periodic holiday visits to the U.S., seemed to be the only course.

Once more the appointment book was examined. One week in February had been set aside to go to a medical conference in Florida. By seeing a few more people each day, I would be able to clear another two weeks. I wrote to Dr. Gordon Thomas that I could come for three weeks. His acceptance was immediate. Thus it was that I found myself on a jet flight from Montreal to Gander, Newfoundland, going northeast to uncertain weather rather than to the sunny south. I had finally broken the shackles that tied me to my practice.

In Gander I had expected an early call from Eastern Provincial Airways, as I had heard that the Grenfell Mission plane, which was transferring patients from small coastal villages to base hospitals on the mainland, would probably be meeting me in Gander the next morning. But I slept in, and I was glad, for I needed the rest after hurrying to finish my work before leaving Toronto. The reason Eastern Airways had not called was soon obvious, as overnight there had been a three-inch snowfall. I was learning my first lesson, that weather is king on the

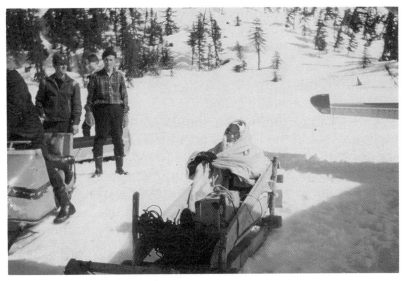

Patient arriving at aircraft on a stretcher (Photo: U. J. Hull).

island. I would lose one day at the beginning.

The next day was beautiful, and I was soon aboard the Eastern's weekly flight to St. Anthony. The DC-3 crossed the islands skirting the ragged coastline and we started dropping as we saw St. Anthony. There waiting with a station wagon was Dr. Walter Spitzer,[4] who had first written to tell me of the need, and his wife Mary Lou, whom I had also known in Toronto. I found myself among friends, including Dr. Gordon Thomas, who had written to me, and Dr. John Gray,[5] the medical specialist. We had met before in 1959, when we had shared a room at a British conference just before John had been married. At that time I had met his fiancée. Later I was to meet her again in their home and see their children.

As I was being guided along the corridor by Dr. Thomas to the room where I was to work I saw a bust of Sir Wilfred Grenfell, and was reminded of a time in 1936 when, as a student in Glasgow University, I listened to him speak during a lunch meeting. I can remember being impressed by his manner and message.

It seemed that I had been drawn to Labrador by a threefold cord—one strand formed in 1963 with Dr. Spitzer's letter, one in 1959 with John Gray and one in 1936 with Wilfred Grenfell.

The hospital was old. The room designated for the eye examination, the occupational therapy room, was the largest available. It was usually called the O.T. room. This was appropriate—I thought the initials should stand for "Odd Things." Outpatients sat in the hallway on a long row of chairs while the clerk took their particulars and hunted for old charts. The ophthalmologist had his own equipment in this room along with an organ covered with drapes and various other items associated with the other uses to which the room was put. Though not always of the latest design, the eye equipment was adequate, with projectochart, lenses, slit lamp and many small but necessary items. Sometimes if there was to be a lecture or discussion group, the eye equipment was moved to one side and chairs brought in. At short notice a visiting priest might want to hold a mass, and then the room changed again to suit this need.

One week was spent in the St. Anthony area, and then the equipment was loaded aboard the Grenfell Mission air ambulance. We were to go to Cartwright, the most northerly nursing station operated from St. Anthony, and back through Forteau, Spotted Island, Port Hope Simpson and Mary's Harbour. As we were only to stay two days in this area, including travelling time, we set to work immediately. Miss Margaret Simms had come to help with the clinic, and the outpatients were ably organized by two station nurses, Misses Greenfield and Chree.

After our stop at the lonely runway near Black Tickle, we landed at Port Hope Simpson. Two patients were waiting for us, brought by dog team and skidoo. The dogs stayed surprisingly quiet, occasionally yawning or licking their chops. The man on the skidoo wanted one of the nurses to visit and check his wife. It meant tying up the plane's busy schedule, but after all, people and problems were what the Mission was all about, and the reason for its existence. Nurse Sheila Chree, who was travelling from Cartwright to replace the nurse at Mary's Harbour, went off on the back of the skidoo. She was soon back

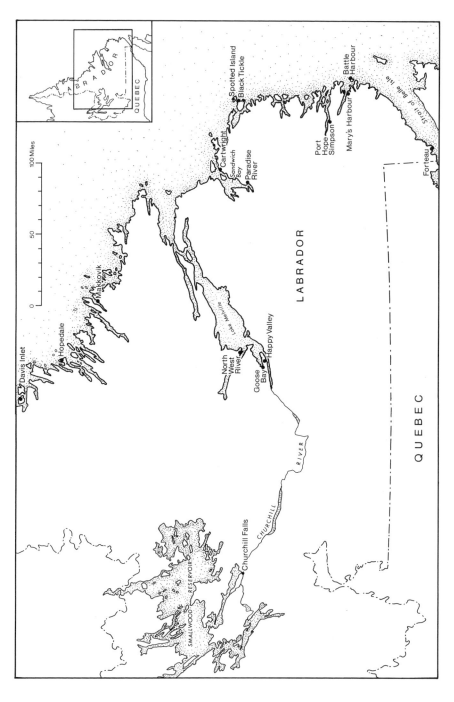

Labrador Coast and Smallwood Reservoir.

and we set off for Mary's Harbour, but a radio message deflected our course to pick up a stretcher case, which we accommodated by shifting the equipment around.

As the stretcher case had to reach St. Anthony as soon as possible the two nurses and I de-planed at Mary's Harbour and in record time removed our equipment. The plane roared away even before we could load a waiting skidoo and qamutiik with our gear.

The trip to Cartwright had gone with precision. Although the setup was much less than with an organized office in Toronto, the mobile equipment was adequate, and reminded me of the days of my early eye training in the 95th British General Hospital in North Africa. The facilities at Mary's Harbour were just about the same, but I was to learn several major lessons there.

The first was that every schedule had the unwritten implication G.W., W.P. (God willing, weather permitting). It was this second factor which was to change the pattern of the trip.

I was to leave the evening of the second day, but it snowed constantly so the plane could not reach us. Fortunately before we packed our equipment the next day we checked with St. Anthony: we were clear but they had the snow. Miss Ruth May, the nurse in charge, was not in the least put out. "Here is the list of second-priority cases—we will call them in today," she instructed.

The next day the weather was still "down" in St. Anthony, so we continued to work our way through the names on our list. I came to understand some of the nuances of language, relics of the time when the early settlers had come from Britain, which made the descriptions of symptoms colourful. One patient was a middle-aged lady who came from Port Hope Simpson. She "found her head"—which meant she had headaches. She was carefully checked. No disease was found to cause the complaint but her glasses were a shocking fit. She had wrapped wool round the frame temples to shorten them so that they looked as if they contained a hearing aid. I told her I could not find anything wrong except the fit of her glasses.

"That's what I thought," she replied. "These glasses were ordered recently during a visit to the capital and this is the way they arrived." As there was no optician on this first trip and we had no suitable temples, we could not adjust her glasses. We measured the length needed, and I suggested she send them back for readjustment. Her reply came in a slow voice. "I thought I would go back to the optician and ask for a job. If he asked what experience I had, I would show him my glasses and tell him no experience seemed to be necessary!" She might have wool behind her ears but no one was going to pull any over her eyes.

Another thing I was to learn at Mary's Harbour was about northern ground transportation. Most of the small outports have roads which surround them, connecting the houses. There may be two or three service trucks to bring goods from the wharf to stores. The nursing station had one such vehicle. For trips between communities, dogsleds were still popular in 1964. Some fear lingered in relation to the new snowmobile which was coming into use. The feeling was that, if travelling alone, the dogs, though slower, would bring you home. The faster snow machines should be used in travelling or hunting in pairs in case of mechanical trouble, or shortage of gas.

The snow that had upset my schedule had also delayed the trip which Nurse Ruth May was to make to the more scattered parts of her district. The slim nurse had now increased her dimension by double layers of garments under a large parka, and so with a guide and a dog team she left for her trip. Miss Chree, who had come from Cartwright with us, took over the station until her return.

The last patient seen and the equipment packed, we awaited the telephone call to tell us that the de Havilland Otter M.I.T. which was to return us to the base at St. Anthony was airborne. The radio phone did ring, but Ruth May broke the news that the weather was down on the Strait of Belle Isle, and it was likely to mean no air transport for some days. We would have to wait, as in winter a plane was the only way from Labrador across the Strait of Belle Isle. If it had been summer, our options would have been greater, as the two following stories illustrate.

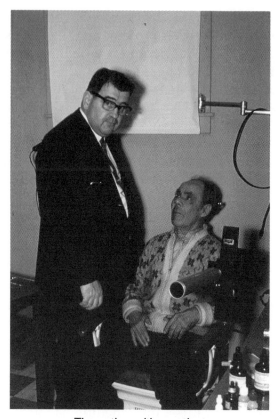

The author with a patient.

On one occasion, I rose to find the summer sky at Mary's Harbour blood red. I ran to fetch my camera to record this scene before it faded. We learned that the plane was grounded by fog in St. Anthony, but, since it was summer, we were able to use the *S.S. Nonia* of the coastal service of the Canadian National Ships, due later in the evening. The local C.N. agent told us that rough seas had held her up a few hours. He advised that we go to bed, to be roused when the ship was approaching.

The call came at 2 a.m. and we were soon whisked to the dock by the mission pick-up. Besides the nurse, Jo Hull, the optician and me, there was also a patient with very advanced cataract, whom we were taking for surgery. She had little more than light perception.

We could see the lights of the *Nonia* anchored in the bay as the tide was very far out. The headlights of our vehicle illuminated the dock, which was otherwise dark. A responding flashlight signal indicated the location of one of *Nonia*'s lifeboats tied up about twenty feet below us. Our equipment was loaded by ropes. Guiding the blind lady into the right position, and supporting her until she could enter the boat was the hard part, but having been a resident of Mary's Harbour for many years she knew what to expect. Finally we were all aboard the launch, and on reaching the *Nonia*, the lifeboat and its contents were lifted to deck level.

Nonia sailed at first light, riding smoothly at first, but when we passed Battle Harbour we reached the rough sea. The dining room started to empty rapidly.

Fortunately Nurse Hull, by contacting the radio operator, was able to speak to the hospital at St. Anthony and arrange transportation to meet us at Cook's Harbour, the first stop the ship made on the island of Newfoundland. To our joy a station wagon was waiting, saving us considerable time and tossing. The *Nonia*, having some other outports to visit, did not reach St. Anthony until later that evening.

Another beautiful morning with a red sky turned into a struggle on a return trip to Paradise River. The eye clinic at the school was originally scheduled to be reached by air, but the plane was needed for other priorities. Miss Greenfield, the nurse in charge, arranged for the services of a local fisherman—the best in Cartwright, she assured me.

We left early, and the sturdy fishing boat made good time down Favourite Tickle into Sandwich Bay, a body of water thirty miles long and about ten miles wide. As Paradise River was near the end of the bay, we had a long way to go. The nurse was waiting to take us to the school. Blankets had been found to pin up on the windows for blackout, and while we set up we were warmed with tea and cake. The school was somewhat basic with an outdoor privy—Joey Smallwood's modernizing had reached only the larger settlements in the 1960s.

We did a session before and after lunch, and the nurse told me that she had worked in the eye department in Moorfields Hospital in London, England before marrying and moving to Labrador. She asked me to send a small modern book for upgrading in latest eye therapy, which I did later.

As we entered Sandwich Bay for the return trip, we found ourselves facing a strong headwind and a cross sea. Reassuringly, the diesel engine throbbed steadily and the fisherman held the course as straight as the corkscrew motion would allow. A skiff attached by a surprisingly fine line bobbed along like a playful dolphin. The optician had found a spray-free corner, wedged between two uprights on deck. After I had watched the headland of Longstretch Point draw no closer after half an hour spent holding on as best I could, it was obvious that our speed had dropped so seriously that we would have a long sail. I decided to explore the cabin.

There was no luxury. An unlit Quebec stove, a mattress-free bunk and some folded blankets made up the fisherman's nest. Borrowing one blanket to rest on and one for my head, I tried to stay as nearly horizontal as possible, with one arm crooked over a metal bar that ran the length of the couch.

Periodically I would ascend to see if our goal was nearer. The smile on the Captain's face was more reassuring than his wind-drowned words: "My boat and I have made it through Sandwich Bay before, we can do it again."

The mariner held his wheel, swaying with the flow, and the optician had settled in to wait it out. This was their sea, and they knew it. Though the sun stayed long in this northern latitude, it had almost set as we turned again into Favourite Tickle. Shielded from the wind it was calmer there, and we made better time. There was a searchlight beam on the boat, but because it used a lot of battery power, the captain used it sparingly to pick up landmarks. Suddenly there were twin beams of light from the shore: someone in a car had heard the beat of our engine. Using its headlights, we were soon tied up, and our equipment and our bodies transferred to the nursing station. The setting sun had not given us a red signal, so we had to wait for the radio forecast.

Long before scientific weathercasting we had learned:

> Red sky at night is the shepherd's delight,
> Red sky in the morning is the sailor's warning.

Sky reading is still used by those whose traditional livelihood depends on the weather, and many will argue their results are more accurate than the new-fangled techniques. The colour of the rising and setting sun was used from time immemorial, and was obviously common in Jesus's time, for He refers to His critics in Matthew 16.2&3: "When evening comes, you say, it will be fair weather for the sky is red, and in the morning it will be stormy for the sky is red and overcast. You know how to interpret the appearance of the sky, but you cannot interpret the signs of the times." The next morning the sun rose without any sanguine hue. The morning "sked" of the plane's movements recorded a trip to Cartwright to pick up the eye team. They made it, and we returned to our base in St. Anthony.

My first clinical visit to Mary's Harbour came to an end with the arrival of the plane. I had not been able to do the work at Forteau as originally planned, but we were in time to share a surprise dinner that was held at the Loon Motel near the St. Anthony airport. The surprise was not for me, but I was happy to share in it. Dr. Gordon Thomas had received a special honour from the Royal College of Surgeons of Canada. The staff of the Grenfell Mission and the townspeople of St. Anthony wanted to share in this, too. With so many involved, it was hard to keep the dinner a secret, but harder still to have all the principals present. Dr. Thomas had to travel frequently, so it was left to Mrs. Thomas to tactfully keep him in St. Anthony. She was assisted in this by a storm which blew up, dumping several feet of snow in the area. But the storm complicated things for Dr. Walter Spitzer, who had been holding clinics in the Roddickton area.[6] He was one of the principals and was to chair the after-dinner program, but there was serious doubt whether he could be back in time. To make matters worse the snow had drifted badly, blocking the road to the Loon Motel. As part of the plan Miss Nichols from Boston, who was on staff of *Deep Sea Fishers*, the International Grenfell Association magazine, and was visiting St. Anthony, invited Dr. and Mrs. Thomas and me to the Loon Motel. By then it had stopped snowing and turned into a lovely evening. Dr. Thomas, as he drove, remarked that he had never seen the road so well-plowed, or so many cars upon it after a storm.

The secret had been well kept, for it was only on arrival that Dr. Thomas realized what had been arranged for him. Only two of the participants were not able to attend, one due to a cancelled flight from Gander and one due to sickness. Dr. Walter Spitzer made it on time. As we introduced each speaker, it was obvious that while the mainland might also honour Dr. Gordon Thomas, he was not without honour among the people who, during the last twenty years, he had served.

While they had a surprise for him, Dr. Thomas also had a surprise for them. A new hospital was to be built in St. Anthony. This would have more beds, more diagnostic and surgical facilities, and departmentalization which would allow specialists to function in their own fields. This, along with an expansion of the air ambulance service, would give St. Anthony a first-class medical facility.

I knew then that somehow I was hooked on the North, and that I would be back to share in the advancing service. What I didn't know then was that I would see the hospital open, and work in it. I would also play a part in designing the layout of the ophthalmological department and its new equipment. The little voice within me had been right.

A new idea is like the rising sun, it catches most people asleep.

Success Diary, February 5, 1980

MY FIRST JOURNEY to Newfoundland had jarred me from my urban-centred life, and made me conscious of the needs of other areas. Not for years had I looked in the "situations vacant" ads in the back of medical journals, but suddenly I became interested in the needs of other zones.

One advertisement interested me. The federal government wanted an ophthalmologist to work for a month in Frobisher Bay[1] on Baffin Island to examine the eyes of school children and deal with eye pathology in the community. Thus it was that in May 1965 I went North once more.

The birds were returning to the Northwest Territories. Many—including the snow bird—travelled from the border of the Antarctic to the sub-Arctic zone around Frobisher Bay. I too was travelling far by winged flight. Four days earlier I had been in Florida with some of my family. On the morning of my departure I was in Toronto, and at noon in Ottawa being briefed by the director of Northern Health Services. After the medical briefing I was handed over to the purchasing agent who had equipment for me to take. That is where my troubles began.

The department in Ottawa had packed three large cartons— including a slit lamp, diagnostic lenses, retinoscope, ophthalmoscope and surgical instruments. These were all supposed to travel with me.

The purchasing agent for the Department of National Health and Welfare, Northern Division, had delivered the cartons to the Ottawa airport, but the express baggage personnel warned him the goods might not be transferred in time to the Nordair flight I was to catch in Montreal. Fortunately he was able to reach me at the department office in Ottawa before I left for the airport, and warn me to make sure the equipment was transferred in Montreal and that I was to ensure it travelled with me. I assured him that I had enough Irish blood in me to see this was done. I did not realize I would need every ounce.

On arrival at Montreal, I reported to the Air Canada freight section and explained that the equipment was being sent up specially for work in the North. It was absolutely essential that it reach the Nordair flight leaving two hours later. After checking at Nordair to present my ticket I went back to Air Canada, but was told they were unable to transfer the equipment. It was not necessary to be bilingual to explain that this was special equipment being sent by the government, and there was absolutely no point in my going North without it. It was finally agreed to make a great concession and bring the shipment to me so I could have it transported to Nordair by red cap service. This was done, and the trouble started all over again.

To begin with, how could they accept special freight at a passenger terminal? Secondly, how could they contact the personnel of the freight section in time? The plane was due to leave in twenty minutes. I was just as obstinate and stubborn as I could be. I was going to talk to the head of Nordair if necessary, and if I did not reach him, I had been told by the federal department to use the Quarantine Medical Service at the airport. I told the clerk the plane would not be leaving without the equipment, even if I had to have the medical officer put a quarantine sticker on it. I was bluffing, of course, but it worked.

The Nordair Super Constellation left late and loaded. A conventional aircraft, it was very noisy compared to the jets now in use. As the sea route to the northern settlements was not yet open, much had to be transported by air. The front part of the cabin up to row twelve had been freed of seats. Sacks of mail, crates and boxes of all sizes—including the three controversial cartons—had been stowed up there. There were also kegs of whisky and a mongrel dog in a crate. Every now and again, when someone annoyed him, he would growl, but on the whole he was very good as air passengers go. He probably did not enjoy the flight or sleep any more than the rest of us.

In forty-eight hours I had travelled nearly 2,000 miles in three different aircraft. I had left the so-called "banana belt" of Florida for Southern Ontario, entered the Arctic Circle and returned to Frobisher Bay. On touching down at 6:20 a.m. I was met by Dr. Mary Habgood, a British graduate of ten years' experience who was medical superintendent of the area and the hospital. During breakfast, I was briefed on the hospital's background and then shown where I was to work. Later I was driven over to the federal building where I was to stay.

After a short rest, I was setting up equipment for the next day's work when a message was received from Broughton Island, about 300 miles north of Frobisher Bay, where there was a little boy with symptoms suggestive of appendicitis. Dr. Habgood informed me that she was going to send a plane to pick him up, and since there were several eye cases on the island, was I interested in making the trip? I was.

After getting clearance on the weather, I found myself airborne about 2 p.m. on a twin-engine Piper Aztec with pilot, navigator and nurse. We headed north across the barren waste of Baffin Island until we could see Cumberland Sound. We flew over an Inuit[2] settlement called Pangnirtung, usually shortened to Pang. After this the scenery became fabulous. The plane threaded its way over low peaks and up fjords where cliffs rose straight out of the sea. One dramatic cliff, about 8,000 feet high, seemed to rise like a skyscraper. We crossed glacier-covered peaks with little green glacial lakes at their base. Then we flew down more fjords which opened onto Davis Strait and landed on a pancake patch of land, Broughton Island, one of the sites on the DEW line.[3]

It would have made quite a picture—two airmen, one nurse, one doctor and multiple Inuit children, all on a large qamutiik covered by a polar bear skin trying to keep our feet off the snow and maintain balance while being pulled by a snowmobile at twenty miles per hour. Unfortunately, I did not have my camera.

Suddenly the engine coughed and stopped. This represented no disaster—the Inuk simply whipped out a wrench, removed the plug, brushed off the points to remove the carbon and replaced it. The snowmobile started and we were on our way.

We then ceremoniously entered the Inuit village, where we collected the patients in a small hostel used as a nursing station. I did a quick external examination of four children and one adult with eye trouble. We decided to take him back with us. He had been hit by a B-B pellet some years before, injuring one eye. His glasses were broken and he was having difficulty seeing with the other eye. We left on our return trip after being entertained by the welfare officer, who also served as medical orderly.

We now had two extra passengers and the wind had changed direction, making the take-off rather hazardous. It seemed certain we were to end our days plowing into one of Baffin's icy mountains, but at the last second, with a steep turn out to sea we gained height and entered the fjords between the fabulous mountains and glacial peaks. We cruised about 190 miles per hour and were soon touching down on the airstrip at Frobisher Bay.

Supper was long over when we reached the hospital, so I was advised to visit the "Blue Kitchen." This sounds like quite a place, but actually consisted of a shack painted blue, an L-shaped counter, one high stool, a hot plate and two refrigerators. I had to have a hot dog because the hamburger patties had not been defrosted. I went back to the federal building and slept.

The federal building was a large structure facing the airstrip. Once the officer's barracks for the United States Strategic Air Command, it cost about $8 million (U.S.) to build but was handed over to the Canadian government for a nominal sum when the U.S. forces pulled out. Now it housed some offices but was mainly reserved for people who, because of the nature of their work, had not set up homes in this northern area. My room on the third floor had a window looking out over the airstrip. Three walls of the room were coloured cream and one was brown. Canary-yellow linoleum covered the floor. Although I had the room to myself there were two beds along with an easy chair, desk, two night tables and good lighting. Toilets and sinks were a hundred yards down the hall, as well as a laundry and shower area with fifteen stalls. It made me feel quite young again, taking me back to my army days.

The hospital was the newest building in Frobisher Bay, having been opened about six months before by the Honourable Judy LaMarsh, federal minister of health. The plans had been laid under the previous administration of the Diefenbaker government. "One sows and another reaps" applies to politics as well as religion. People and problems persist but politicians pass, so it is only right for them to attract what glory they can in their hour upon the stage.

The hospital had thirty-five beds, a good operating room and a cafeteria which served good meals. It also had three doctors although one, Dr. Drabitt, was on leave. The hospital had no designated eye room, so the longest and largest room we could find was commandeered. The days in the army had taught scrounging, so as many tables and chairs as could be found soon provided the elements of a waiting room. A dental chair of venerable age with foot-pedal pump action was found and dusted off. The lens box, trial frame and slit lamp were quite old, but functional. We set up the screen and projection equipment, using blankets to separate the waiting room from the examination area. Presto—the clinic was ready!

I worked a month in Frobisher Bay, mainly screening school children, both Inuit and Caucasian who sat side-by-side with the same lighting and using the same textbooks in the school house, the only one in the settlement. Here was an excellent opportunity to work on the problem of myopia. The children could be examined with baselines as nearly as possible the same. Living conditions and diet, however, were not comparable. There had been some discussion in medical circles suggesting that the refractive status of the two groups was quite different. In this test, where the children were examined class by class, with the same age groups and illumination in each class, I found that the percentage of long- and short-sighted children was exactly the same. There are some who feel that these figures are not really representative, since Caucasians have settled so long in the larger communities in the North that there remain no pure-blooded Inuit except in the most isolated settlements.

Many of the white settlers were very transient, like me, coming to do special jobs for short periods of time and staying in residences or in the newer part of the town near the airport. The great oil storage tanks, which had to keep the community running through the long winter months, the R.C.M.P., school and Anglican church were all closely huddled at the harbour, as if for warmth and support. Most of the Inuit lived in Apex, about three miles from the harbour, and there the Hudson's Bay Company had its store. There too lived the soapstone carvers, some very expert at their art.

Halfway up the hilly road between the settlements was the hospital. Modern and functional in its design, the architect had not forgotten aesthetics, since on the outer wall was a design of an Inuit with sled and dogs.

It seemed the residents of the North and the short-term visitors from the south worked and played well together. The North, with its harsh weather, develops a warmth in its residents toward one another. One such relaxation period was called "Toonik Time," when competitions of all sorts were run on the still-frozen harbour. We had a visitor that year, the Honourable John G. Diefenbaker, who with his wife, Olive, toured the hospital. A platform had been set up on a small frozen lake beside the road to Apex. While some played broom ball, others released balloons of many colours and a small crowd slowly gathered. Although about 9 p.m. it was still bright in the land of the midnight sun. John Diefenbaker arrived, made a short speech, which was wise as it was turning chilly, and started to mingle with people. Everyone knew of his particular interest in the North and wanted to shake his hand. Clad in a sealskin coat, he stood head and shoulders above the average parka-clad Inuit.

No one seemed sure who the Toonik were, but the Inuit associate them with the blond giants who lived in the North before the present natives came. Perhaps they had the idea that

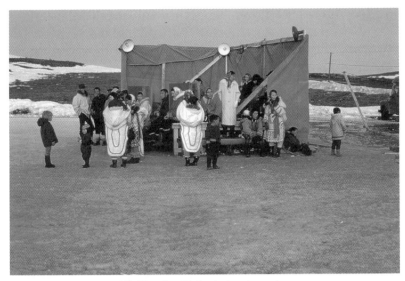

Waiting for Diefenbaker to arrive.

evening that one of the Toonik had returned on this special day—a giant of a man—John Diefenbaker.

I learned a great deal when I was in Frobisher Bay. Since there was no television I found the library stimulating. I learned the wasteland beyond the small hills around Frobisher Bay was really teeming with life, some of it hidden and hibernating through the winter, but in the spring stirring with new activity.

Spring was bursting all over that part of the Arctic, with the sun rising at 2 a.m. and setting at 10 p.m. The sun here has a long day, trying to remove the chill from the North for twenty continuous hours. The glare of the sun reflected from the snow was so intense that dark glasses were mandatory, and colour photography required special filters. With the thermometer swinging between twenty-five and fifty degrees Fahrenheit, the continuous white sheet of snow rolled slowly backwards revealing dark patches of earth, rock and low scrubby bushes. There were no trees. Even the hardy varieties which could live in the thin layer of soil covering the rock over so much of Newfoundland could not survive the cold and penetrating wind of Frobisher Bay.

Birds which had flown south during the winter and returned were making new nests. The Inuit who had been trapping furbearing animals (which now had the best and thickest pelts) were about to reap the rewards in fur actions of their strenuous labour.

Freight-bearing planes were refuelling, as a rich body of ore had been found further north and bulldozers and construction gear were being massed for the development. Students were on their way to the icefields as part of the glacier watch, mapping the movement of these giants. Soon the harbour would be a hive of activity as the ice left the bay and the supply ships moved in. What had not been carefully planned and ordered ahead would have to wait for another year. The short three-month shipping season was just long enough for one trip.

I learned about bureaucracy in Frobisher Bay. My experience with Revenue Canada was only as a contributor, a common taxpayer. Now I was to find out what the tax structure was supporting. When I had been a government employee previously, it was in the British army during World War II. If things were not right it was easy to say, "There's a war on, what can you expect?" Now there was an army of civil servants in peace-time working hard in our interest. But still our roof leaked!

On returning from the hospital one evening I found that another room had been assigned to me. Snow on the flat roof was melting rapidly, and a stream of water had come down soaking my former bed, but fortunately the cupboard where my personal things were stored suffered no damage. Apart from the inconvenience of moving to another room, no harm was done. I was told the roof had leaked the year before and application for the necessary roofing supplies had gone to Ottawa. Unfortunately, the forms had been too-long delayed in transit from one desk to another. It was believed that the supplies had missed the boat, and would probably take another year.

Every day on my way to work I passed the Department of Transport yard which had vehicles waiting for parts to be sent up by air from Montreal. I had noticed that the Department of Transport used General Motors vehicles and the Navy used

Chrysler Corporation. The Department of Health, with its idea of service to all, had a Jeep, one Fargo van, and one Ford Fairlane with an automatic transmission. This latter, without four-wheel drive, was out of commission the whole month I was there. The Fargo also had problems but the Jeep, the oldest of the three, kept on going. Why, I wondered, could not one make of vehicle be used in each settlement in the Arctic—Ford in one, Chrysler in another and so on. This would mean that only one automaker's spare parts would keep the settlement mobile, and spares from scrapped vehicles would keep the others running. "That would never work," I was told. "Each department budgets and purchases its own vehicles in Ottawa." The Department of Transport could have the headache, and the taxpayer the expense of air transportation for parts.

Bureaucracy was also evident in the medical field. Among my patients I found some who had strabismus, or "turn" in the eye, which required surgical intervention. Surely with a fine new hospital and operating room, we could do the operation here. I had the expertise and the instruments. All that was needed was an anaesthetist. As the giving of anaesthetics to children for eye muscle surgery requires some extra care and training, I felt it would be good to have a specialist in this field come North for two days, especially as the hospital was understaffed. It was explained to me that this was simply not done. The normal method was for children to be evacuated to Montreal where they were placed in foster homes and assessed in eye outpatient departments of hospitals. They then returned to the foster homes until the surgery could be performed. After discharge they returned to the foster homes, being checked by the outpatient clinics until they could return to the North. All this could take a month or more and cost a great deal of money. Besides the expense, it seemed to me immoral to take Inuit children into strange and often-frightening surroundings for such an elective surgical procedure. This emotional trauma could probably be more damaging than the original condition.

After my protests, it was decided that if I could find an anaesthetist who would come up North they would pay his expenses and a fee. I rang Toronto, and through the good

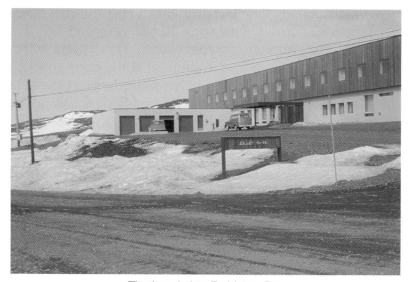

The hospital at Frobisher Bay.

offices of Dr. Nelles Silverthorne, president of the Christian Medical Society, an anaesthetist who was taking time off for study came up. We met him at 2:30 a.m. and, after resting, he was able to function about noon. We operated upon four cases that afternoon and four the next morning. He was able to instruct the resident staff in the finer points of the use of the new anaesthetic equipment before he left that evening. While in hospital the Inuit children could have visits from their family and could quickly return to their care. I followed them during the rest of my stay and Dr. John Speakman, who visited Frobisher Bay later that year on the regular call of the medical supply ship *C.D. Howe*, was able to see them in their final healed state. A great deal of money in airfares and in foster home expense was saved. Better still, the children had not been taken from their home town to a new and alien environment.

Now that I had leaped this hurdle, I thought that progress would be rapid toward the goal of providing better service for the North through cooperation with the academies of medicine in the large centres. With this in mind, I made up a statement under the title "Canada's Northland is Challenging You."[4] I wished to make the point that the Northwest Territories was a federal responsibility and therefore a challenge to all Canadian doctors, no matter to what province they belonged. I had noticed that the care of northern people, medical and nursing, was being carried out mainly by professionals trained outside Canada. The two doctors in Frobisher Bay were trained in the U.K. and most of the nurses in the outstations were from Britain, the Commonwealth, or even Spain. This was because Canadian nurses were not regularly given training in obstetrics, while the others were. This meant that Canadian nurses had to be used in the hospital service only. Comments of this kind, although truthful, were not appreciated by the bureaucracy of the Canadian Medical Association, which would not publish my article. I finally gave it to the Grenfell Mission magazine *Among the Deep Sea Fishers*, where it appeared in the July 1966 edition (reprinted in this volume as Appendix D). My approach to the C.M.A. editorial top brass had not been successful. I had been too impatient.

While much of the work on the trip to Frobisher Bay was routine, there were some parts which were scientifically stimulating. Two areas were particularly profitable for study. One was myopia, the other phlyctenulosis. The ophthalmologist previously hired by the federal government to survey the North was Dr. Elizabeth Cass.[5] She had expressed concern in her reports about these two areas, and suggested that phlyctenulosis was an early sign of exposure to the tubercle bacillus. Indeed, the incidence of tuberculosis was high in northern inhabitants, but the specialists in respiratory diseases did not agree that phlyctenulosis was only due to this cause.

The investigation of myopia was important as three theories were current at that time. Elizabeth Cass's strongly held view that the change in diet, from the use of the natural food of the hunter and gatherer to that shipped in from the south, was the cause. This was hard to accept as the only reason. For one thing, when game became scarce, people gathered in communities instead of being nomadic. About the same time—as the language of the northern peoples was being reduced to writing—schools were being built where English was taught, and electric lighting was being installed. Theory two held that the near work associated with the schools, and the new lighting were the real factors. Theory three held that external factors were only incidental, and that genetic determination of the shape of the face was the cause. The more elongated Caucasian faces were more inclined to hyperopia (long-sightedness), while the rounded features of Mongolian faces were more associated with myopia (short-sightedness).

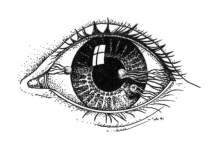

Phlyctenular ulcers.
(Sketch by Dr. J. Watt.)

With my captive subjects in the schools consisting of both these groups, whom I had to examine anyway, it seemed an excellent time to study this third hypothesis. As my visit to Frobisher Bay was ending I analyzed the figures. Taking the spherical equivalent of each eye separately, I found I had refracted 271 persons (542 eyes) of which 189 had Mongolian features and 82 were of Caucasian extraction. On checking the 378 Mongolian and the 164 Caucasian eyes I was surprised to find that long-sighted and short-sighted eyes appeared in the same percentage in each group. As the time was too short and the series too small, I never published these findings except in my report to the federal government. My own feeling is that all three theories have merit, and all play some part in the visual acuity of northern residents.

During my routine examinations I found that some patients had extreme difficulty facing the light. This photophobia is a telltale sign that there is an active process on the cornea. On closer inspection, a leash of blood vessels can be revealed tracking across the conjunctiva, ending at one or two blisters at the junction of the white sclera and the clear cornea. This is a typical picture of the phlycten, and on healing this produces a scar. If several episodes of phlyctenulosis have occurred, the cornea will be thinned and irregular enough to reduce vision.

In the 189 Inuit cases, six of the patients had the disease in active form. In one case, the cornea was so thin that I was afraid it would perforate, as had some of the badly scarred cases I had seen. While I agreed that this disease represented an immune reaction, I felt that the shortage of naturally occurring vitamin C so characteristic of northern winters might have a triggering effect. This idea is further developed in my article "The Cornea in Canada's Northland" (reprinted in this volume as Appendix E). For the case with the very thin cornea, I used the only vial I could find of injectable ascorbic acid. This, along with local sulpha drops, produced a marked reduction in the photophobia, and the cornea started to heal.

While one case proves little, it is important to realize that, especially after a long winter has reduced blood levels of vitamin C, sudden saturation to normal levels can turn the therapeutic corner. It is also important to realize that steroids for use in the eye in drops or ointment were not readily available in the Arctic in 1965.

Meanwhile Dr. Elizabeth Cass, who had previously worked in the eastern Arctic, had moved to the western Arctic and found the Indian and Metis in that region hardly different from those in the east. Dr. Lyall Black of the federal Department of Health was constantly bombarded with her reports and requests for more help. Whether my month-long survey at Frobisher Bay was the only response he could make within his narrow budget, I do not know.

Nevertheless Dr. Cass was to find a larger international forum, for I heard her speak at the Pan-American Association of Ophthalmology in Montreal in 1966.[6] This was followed by papers in Munich, Germany, and an article in the *Canadian Journal of Ophthalmology* in 1973 entitled "A Decade of Northern Ophthalmology."[7] With this negative exposure of Canadian ophthalmology in the North, some response from the university establishment was mandatory. Armed with a grant from Health and Welfare, a survey team headed by Dr. R. W. Morgan, professor and chairman, Department of Preventive Medicine, University of Toronto was sent North. This was followed in February 1974 by an ophthalmology team which flew into Gjoa Haven and Spence Bay. These two communities were chosen as being least affected by white influence and genes.

These endeavours resulted in an article, "Inuit myopia: an environmentally induced 'epidemic?'."[8] More articles were to appear, so that the Canadian Ophthalmological Society had to run a special, extra-thick journal called the *Symposium on Arctic Ophthalmology*.[9] Though much needling had been necessary, the pachydermatous skin of the federal and medical bureaucracy had finally been pierced to recognize people with need in the North.

Today the winds have changed. There is now some link between Memorial University in St. John's, Newfoundland and the Labrador Coast; between McGill University in Montreal and Frobisher Bay, Kingston and Moosonee, the University of Toronto and Sioux Lookout, and the University of Manitoba and Churchill. Calgary has a student affiliation with Yellowknife, while the University of Alberta in Edmonton sends professionals to Inuvik, and the University of British Columbia also extends its care to the northland. I should have remembered that a seed must be buried before it sprouts, or as Jesus Christ said: "Except a kernel of wheat fall into the ground and dies, it remains only a single seed. But if it dies it produces many seeds." (John 12. 24) Ideas are the same. They may be buried for five years or more but then suddenly germinate. I should have learned another lesson in the North—there is always motion, even in the giant glaciers. Bureaucracy may seem fearsome and cold but if carefully watched and charted, progress is being made.

During the time that I was in Baffin, I was to meet a youth who, in my opinion, was one of the most fortunate I have ever seen. A call had come from Grise Fiord, the most northerly of the Inuit settlements, to say that there had been a head injury in a hunting camp ("on the land," the Inuit call it) about a two-hour dog sled ride from the nursing station. Dr. Mary Habgood had to make a difficult decision—should she charter a DC-3 for a flight which would take at least five hours each way, perhaps to find the boy already dead, or should she wait a little? Mary shared the problem with me, probably knowing of my years in the army during World War II. I advised temporization until a report reached her from Grise Fiord. If he reached there alive, he would make it on the long second leg of the journey: resuscitation at the nursing station would be better than hasty evacuation.

I saw the teenager next morning and found him in much better physical and mental condition than I would have expected for one who had a gunshot wound to the head. A 22-calibre rifle had discharged during cleaning and the bullet had penetrated through the soft tissue just behind the lower jaw in the midline. There was an exit wound through his tongue and another in the forehead between the root of the nose and the hairline.

With the tongue injured, it was difficult for him to speak, but I was able to ascertain that he could read 20/30 in the right and 20/40 in the left eye. Dilation of the pupils revealed that while there was some bruising of the retina, there was no gross haemorrhage and no penetration of either eyeball. How the bullet had escaped both eyeballs and the chiasma where the optic nerves cross was a cause of great wonderment.

In view of so much tissue damage near the brain and the nature of the watery discharge from the nose, we felt that he should not only be "covered" by what antibiotics we had, but referred to a teaching centre to have further assessment.

The next day, the phone rang. It was the resident from Montreal. Did we not know better than to send a case for plastic reconstruction without an appointment? We explained that the case was sent because we thought that there might be a leakage of cerebrospinal fluid, which we could not exclude. Did he not receive our letter of request for admission?

Long before the youth returned to the Arctic, I had left Frobisher Bay, so I did not hear the ultimate findings. Another part of the story was to unfold later in Roddickton, Newfoundland. After the clinic was over, there was nothing to do after the evening meal, which tended to be prolonged. As is usual when medical personnel spend time together, there is much shop talk. I recounted the above story, speaking of the boy as the luckiest fellow I had ever seen, when a voice from the other end of the table said "I was the nurse at Grise Fiord when that boy was brought in and sent him on to you." Like many others who service the North, her stay had not lasted until the return of the patient, so she could add little. Some of the senior members of the nursing staff of the Grenfell organization had stayed to make it a life's work, but most who served the remote places had short terms.

Another thing that gives pleasure in retrospect is that Dr. West, one of the resident physicians who assisted at surgery during my northern trip, is now an ophthalmologist. Apparently he was looking for a specialty that would give him satisfaction. So a seed dropped in a remote hospital and watered by Dr. Speakman, who visited two months later, brought into bloom a colleague now practising 5,000 miles away from the original sowing. Dr. West practices ophthalmology on Vancouver Island.

3 / The Impact of Grenfell and Smallwood on Northern Settlers

> We make an income from what we get, but we make a life from what we give.
>
> *Winston Churchill*

NEWFOUNDLANDERS HAVE a knack for giving optimistic and hopeful names to places, some of which do not warrant the description. One such name is "Strait of Belle Isle," which should have been called "Killer Narrows."

Belle Isle is situated at the apex of the bottle-shaped Gulf of St. Lawrence as if it were a champagne cork. Mute evidence of the danger of the narrows hangs in the foyer of the new Grenfell Hospital at St. Anthony, just around the tip of the peninsula, in the form of the crest of one of Her Majesty's ships picked up along the shore. This crest tells of long-ago tragedy, probably before the lighthouse was built in 1854.

Much earlier in Newfoundland's history, there was so much rivalry and war between the great maritime powers—Britain, France, Spain and Portugal—that little settlement was allowed. It was desired to keep Newfoundland as a fishing base, with no year-round residents. Nevertheless small communities developed; the northern peninsula indicates the influence of French and British settlers, the Spanish and Portuguese codfishery remaining mainly in the south. Typical French names dot the east side: Quirpon, Griquet, Croque and Conche; while Boat Harbour, Cook's Harbour, Eddies Cove, Savage Cove, and Flower's Cove occupy the peninsula opposite the Labrador coast.

There was some contact with the Beothuk Indians—possibly the name Savage Cove signifies this. When the first white fishermen settled in numbers there were clashes sparked mainly by the different attitudes to property. The Beothuks, like most

Indian tribes, held goods in common, so if they found fishing or hunting gear they thought nothing of borrowing it. If this belonged to a European, the culprit was immediately accused of stealing, and though they were excellent archers, their primitive archery was no match for the guns of the new arrivals. Later, the hatred became so intense that to kill a native was considered a feat of arms to be noted as an exploit. The Beothuks never learned how to handle guns, or they might have been able to defend themselves against the French-armed MicMac Indians, who hunted them as savagely as the whites.

It had not always been so, for in 1612 John Guy had established friendly relations with the Beothuks, and promised to return. When a ship came in sight at the promised time, the natives, thinking that Guy had kept his promise, crowded the shore. Unfortunately, it was another captain who mistook the group as hostile, and fired. The natives, thinking this was treachery on Guy's part, feared the white man's killer stick and perfidy.

Slavery was in its heyday, and many were taken this way. The Portuguese navigator Gaspar de Corte Real was identified as a trader, but French and Spaniards were also involved in slave-running. The Beothuk men (some of whose skeletons have been found) were over six feet tall and probably fetched a good price.

As more coves were filled with immigrants, around the coast the noose was tightening on the remaining Beothuks, who survived by fishing on the Exploits River and Red Indian Lake in their twenty-foot birchbark canoes, and by killing what deer they could find. A story by Harold Horwood[1] tells of fighting which erupted between small French settlements and the Indians, and in the ensuing battle the French were wiped out at St. Julien's, Grandois and Croque. One of the fishermen in Conche told me he had picked up so many arrowheads he thought there must have been a battle there. Not realizing the import to archaeology or history, he had sold them cheaply to visitors.

There are few, if any, pockets of French language left on the peninsula, but the Roman Catholicism brought by the early sett-

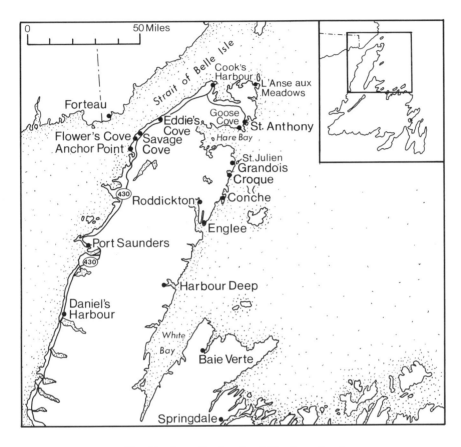

The Northern Peninsula of Newfoundland.

lers remains strong among settlers on the east side—Conche being entirely Roman Catholic though Englee, slightly further south, is strongly Pentecostal.

Frederick Rowe[2] gives us one of the main reasons for Anglo dominance in Newfoundland—economic necessity. Countries on the mainland of Europe had access to salt deposits, while England did not. This meant their codfishery was dealt with in different ways. The French and Spanish could preserve their fish with salt and sail to their home ports. The English had to slit, clean and dry the fish on "flakes." This required shore space and considerable time and skill, as well as a great deal of handling. At times this could not be completed by the departure date and some men may have been left ashore.

Another reason for settling developed from the brutality of the fishing admirals. Conditions on the ships could be so intolerable that those set ashore to locate fresh water or wood simply stayed. Gradually, little pockets of settlement developed in bays along the coasts. As the admirals arrived in May and left in September, there was no law for eight months of the year. Second-generation settlers, when asked who they were, replied they were "Liveyeres" (because "we live 'ere"); others have called them "Jackatars."

The origin of English settlers on the west side of the peninsula has been researched by the Institute of Social and Economic Research at Memorial University,[3] some of which can be relayed. The first settler on the northern part of the coast was Robert Bartlett, who arrived at Anchor Point about 1740. He and a companion had left a ship in White Bay to get some wood but had been captured by Indians, who made them carry their burdens. At night, while the Indians slept around their campfire, they escaped. Whether this story is true, or fabricated as a means of combating a charge of desertion, is uncertain. They travelled across the northern peninsula to Anchor Point, where they found an American schooner whose crew was "making fish." Bartlett decided to settle there, and sent his companion back to England with a message summoning his nephew to this area of plentiful fish, seal, game and wild fruit. He was joined the next year by one nephew and by another a few years later. This latter, Abram Genge, became a leader. When joined by other Englishmen and Scots, he hired them and designated to each an area of coast. The fish and furs he collected were taken by American schooners.

Up to this time there were no women on the coast, but they were to be supplied by the Watts family. Watts worked for Genge for a time, and had two sons and two daughters. The first daughter married a man named William Buckle, and from them sprang all the Buckles in Labrador. The second daughter, Mary, married a Lieutenant Duncan, who deserted from one of His Majesty's ships. To escape the authorities he changed his name to Gould, his mother's name. This occurred between 1795 and 1800, and the union produced fourteen children, only three of them boys. The eleven girls, all beautiful, became wives for the men scattered in small communities with such names as Savage Cove, Black Duck Cove and Eddies Cove.

With the difficulty of travel by sea in the winter and of walking over rough terrain, the regular courting patterns of young swains was limited to approximately ten miles. Consanguinity arose inevitably, and this was to produce some of the medical problems and congenital defects which complicated the work of Wilfred Grenfell, who was the first to bring organized medical care to the area. Grenfell's first voyage aboard the *S.S. Albert* was in 1892, when the sea was the only significant highway to and around Newfoundland.

Grenfell was a doctor with a high sense of adventure, and with a driving energy fed by his firm Christian faith. I heard Sir Wilfred, as he had then become, tell his story in 1936, the year he retired from medical practice. He was a lunch speaker at Glasgow University, where I was studying medicine. I had heard stories of this romantic yet humanitarian figure who had devoted his life to seamen, particularly those who lived in appalling conditions on the coast of Newfoundland and Labrador. I had expected a man as big as his reputation, but as he ascended the platform I saw a spare old man of medium height and athletic figure. He spoke simply but compellingly.

I listened spellbound as he told how his life had been changed from one of drifting to one of purpose by attending a meeting addressed by D. L. Moody, a U.S. evangelist. Wilfred had wanted to respond to the message Moody had delivered, but held back until he saw a young naval midshipman rise in the midst of his peer shipmates. Knowing how much courage must have been required to face the ribbing and abuse of his shipmates, Wilfred also accepted the challenge to confess his faith. Although known for making rapid—even rash—decisions, this was one that Grenfell would never regret.

Probably through his father's connection with the London Hospital, young Wilfred came to know Sir Fredrick Treves, a keen Christian and one of the foremost surgeons of his time. He decided to enter medicine, and after his graduation Treves, who was on the board of the Mission to Deep Sea Fishermen, recruited young Grenfell to be a surgeon on a ship attending the fishing fleet on the North Sea. This allowed Wilfred to fulfil his two greatest loves simultaneously—that of God and the sea.

While all fishing in those days was laborious and full of maiming and fatal accidents, reports were reaching the Mission that conditions off the coast of northern Newfoundland were much worse. Grenfell was sent to investigate and help. After a long, rough journey the little ship *Albert* entered the harbour at St. John's just as a great fire had broken out in the city. Nevertheless he was able to obtain enough supplies to sail 1,000 miles north as far as Hopedale on the Labrador coast, treating 900 fishermen and the "Liveyeres" who stayed year-round in primitive shacks.

I was only twenty-one years old at the time I heard him speak. Adventure and challenge were high on my priorities, as they had been for Grenfell. I listened with fascination as he told a story of his near death when marooned on an iceberg in Hare Bay with his dog team. His voice was thick with emotion as he told of sacrificing three dogs whom he had come to love. He fashioned a rug and coat from their hides, and used the carcasses as a windbreak. The other dogs he induced to curl up beside him so their bodies kept him warm. Exhausted and cold he fell asleep, placing his care in God's hands. On waking he found that the icepan had left the bay, and was nearer the point behind which St. Anthony nestled. He dissected the long bones from the dogs to make a makeshift pole, and used his shirt as a flag.

Meanwhile four men who had been skinning seals on the headland saw that something strange was happening at sea. The only telescope in St. Anthony was located, and the object scrutinized. It was surmised that this was their doctor, who had raced off to see a sick patient on the other side of the bay and had not been heard of since.

I had no way of knowing then that nearly thirty years later I would actually be in St. Anthony and have an elderly patient tell me he had been the one to see the spot on the sea, and had been one of the rescue team. I did not know that I would actually stay at Grenfell House and view the plaque which Wilfred had dedicated to the dogs who had died to save his life—Moody, Watch, and Spy.

Grenfell's work has now been recognized in the educational as well as the medical field. I quote from *The Development of Education in Newfoundland* by Frederick W. Rowe, who was once minister of education in the cabinet of Premier Smallwood:

> Following the pattern he had set in his medical work, Grenfell was able to induce large numbers of volunteer teachers from the American colleges and schools to come to northern Newfoundland and Labrador and conduct schools during the summer session. In addition to the seasonal schools four "mission schools" were established at St. Anthony, St. Mary's River, Cartwright and North West River. These schools not only provided education for the local inhabitants but with their dormitories made it possible for children from the small communities, where no schools existed, to board the year round at the mission schools.[4]

Rowe also gives tribute to the International Grenfell Association in its connections with the U.S. and Canadian colleges, which were able to provide grants and bursaries for the better students in the North, so that those in previously neglected areas often obtained better education than the average city child in Newfoundland.

Wilfred Grenfell had come to the "Liveyeres" in the coves with a healing touch and a message. Up until then their greatest achievement had been the ability to survive. Those who were born on the coast, especially in the winter, had a particularly hard time as the fishing fleet sailed south for eight months of the year.

Births were aided by whomever was available, frequently under primitive, unsanitary conditions. As often the mother was undernourished or diseased, the chance of the baby living until the sun rose high and the ice departed was low. Tuberculosis was rampant in both adults and children. The essential nature of vitamins was unknown, and without naturally occurring vitamin C in the winter months scurvy was a dangerous threat. The people had not learned what the Inuit had long ago discovered—that uncooked seal meat retains its anti-scorbutic power but that it is destroyed in the cooking. Only those with enough wisdom and foresight to have retained summer berries or edible green plants could escape the terrible scourge of those who wintered in the Arctic.

For the strong who survived the early days, the hazards of outport fishing were also very real. Children went with their fathers on the small boats as early as seven years of age, and shared the risk of crippling injury or drowning. The water is so deep along most of the coast that there are few areas where a young child could learn to swim, so most of the fishermen had never learned this life-saving skill.

Long before the words or the music were written, "You're nobody till somebody loves you," Grenfell knew that was the answer. So he came to those who felt abandoned, shut off from the rest of the world for eight months of the year, with the message that God loved them. Because they were people whom his Master loved, Wilfred Grenfell loved them too. As others, similarly motivated, also came to stay on the coast to care for them through the long hard winters, people began to believe in themselves. Besides his medical work, the formation of the cooperatives and the schools were all designed to emphasize the fact that they were people who were worth more than they were receiving, and there was no reason for them to be exploited or neglected any more.

Twenty-five years were to pass after Grenfell's death on October 9, 1940 before I was to join the team of professionals who were continuing his work, and very dramatic changes had occurred.

I have heard criticisms that Dr. Grenfell, who had formed a mission to help the people in the northern peninsula and Labrador, spent his time during the winter months in Britain, the United States and Canada. This statement, though true, completely misses the fact that the only way in which the work could survive was through fund-raising. To have tried to run, far less to develop the work from local resources would have been impossible.

The winter months were the time when lecture tours could be profitable, and recruits, who were required more and more as the mission grew, could be contacted. His was the mind of the architect who could see the great design and could sell it to others. Money flowed in, but it was soon apparent that he was not talented as a draughtsman or expense accountant. It was a fortunate day when Grenfell severed his connection with the National Mission to Deep Sea Fishermen, which he had joined in 1888, and the International Grenfell Association was registered in 1914. This organization allowed him to do what he did best, lecture tours in the winter, and sailing into the coves along the rugged coast to help the sick and needy in the summer, when he could fit into the lives of those who had been isolated during the winter. He visited a string of nursing stations, which were open all year around, and schools, which operated during the summer, but these were mostly about 200 miles apart.

While much of the North was benefiting from the money raised, opposition in St. John's, where the government and the merchants were, was growing. Newfoundlanders are proud people and some felt that in his lecture tours Grenfell had slurred the government and the economy of Newfoundland by telling outsiders of its serious financial need. He was impeached but vindicated on all charges in 1914.

Eight years after Grenfell had arrived in the North, a child was born in Gambo, who was to have as great an impact on the whole of the island as Grenfell had had on Labrador: his name was Joseph Smallwood. Through his writing of the book *I Chose Canada*, we learn that while things had been bad before, the economy in the Depression years from 1929 on was disastrous in the extreme, and he decided to do something about it. His description of the economic and health conditions prevalent at that time could not be better given than in his own writing.

In the United States, across Canada, and in Newfoundland, the same word was employed to describe the amount of unemployment, poverty, disease, and hunger there was in each country: depression. But it was totally incongruous to use the same word to describe the wildly different conditions in the three countries. In Newfoundland, depression meant hunger, real hunger; hunger for over half the population; hunger that left people hungry day after day, for months, for years; hunger that so weakened families that their resistance to disease was reduced close to the minimum. Many of the men who were fortunate enough to get jobs in the pulp and paper companies' logging camps came in ravenously hungry and had to eat for two and three weeks before they put enough flesh back on their bones to be able to swing a bucksaw again. The report of the Canadian medical team that investigated the state of people's health in superbly beautiful Bonne Bay shocked us all. We were all of us frightened of tuberculosis, suspicious of neighbours and friends—and relatives—afraid to get X-ray photographs taken of our lungs, and afraid not to. We had the highest incidence of tuberculosis to be found anywhere north of the Mexican border. We also had the highest rates of infant mortality, maternal mortality (deaths of mothers in childbirth), and contagious, infectious, and otherwise communicable diseases in North America. The one-third of our people who were on the six cents a day, $1.80 a month, dole deteriorated visibly in health, for the dole was simply not enough to sustain life.[5]

After heavy and difficult campaigning over some years, Smallwood was able to arrange a confederation with Canada in 1949. He became the first Liberal Premier of Newfoundland and set about to develop the resources and to improve the health of the people.

When I arrived in Newfoundland in 1964, highways and hospitals were either completed or being built. The Trans-Canada Highway was being paved, and new hospitals were being built in the central area of Newfoundland at Grand Falls and Gander. Relations between the International Grenfell Association and the Smallwood administration were excellent throughout "Joey's" term in office, and the new hospital at Happy Valley to honour Dr. Harry Paddon had just been erected.

"Expand or perish" had been one of the themes of Smallwood's campaigns, and he was concerned that so many of Newfoundland's youth were going to the mainland for training and work. It was therefore appropriate that in 1949, on the first Speech from the Throne after Confederation, he announced that Memorial College, which had been formed in honour of the dead of World War I, would be upgraded to a degree-granting university forthwith. By 1966, enrollment was to grow from an initial 307 to 4,762 students. In 1964, during my time of visiting Newfoundland, Lord Brain came from Britain as a consultant and advised in favour of the establishment of a medical school. In 1969, the Memorial University Medical School was opened, and in 1973 its first medical doctors graduated.[6] The Charles Curtis Memorial Hospital in St. Anthony, which had been promised by Joey Smallwood in 1964 and was officially opened May 30, 1968, became an associated teaching facility of the university medical school. Dr. Gordon Thomas, director of the hospital, was appointed professor of surgery, and Dr. John Gray, chief of medicine at the hospital, was appointed assistant professor of medicine.

Road routes to reach the base hospital were expanding too, as a road ran to St. Anthony from the Trans-Canada Highway, near Deer Lake. In the summer, the unpaved road was usually kept well-graded, but using it in the winter had its hazards, as I well remember from one bad trip from Grand Falls in January, 1969.

Had I been more superstitious, I would have been warned by the mysterious smashing of a side mirror on the camper van in which I transported my equipment. Then I slipped on the frozen path outside my office and had to have stitches on the skin over my elbow. As I was not too disabled and I was travelling with the optician, Ross Fraser, who could do most of the driving, we set off.

The problems on this trip were far from over, for just a few miles short of Deer Lake, we ran out of fuel. With the help of a passing motorist, we were able to reach our destination. The vehicle had been cold, and we found out as we filled up with gasoline that our radiator was low. The service station was out of antifreeze, so we had to use water. Turning northward, we passed Bonne Bay, appropriately named, for even in winter it is beautiful.

The gravel road was ploughed, but "skiddy" at time, and we had to dig out twice. We had only one shovel, and as Ross was much younger than I, and my elbow was still troublesome, he had the longer spells of digging. We had also multiple stops, as our radiator kept becoming low, and the red light in the engine came on. We, of course, had to wait for cooling and then try to fill up the radiator with snow—a most unsatisfactory procedure. Further along, we found a running stream and so used our thermos flasks, long since emptied, to help our need. In the process, my foot slipped into the stream and the cup of the thermos floated away. Fortunately, I had extra socks and shoes in the van. Ross, a native Newfoundlander from Bishop's Falls, was used to making light of difficulty, but we were both in need of something to make us laugh. Suddenly it hit us at the same time: the best "buckets" we could have for filling the radiator were the rubber boots that I had just removed!

By the time we reached Daniel's Harbour, it was time for a refill and a refreshment stop. We were now hopelessly behind schedule, and so we rang the nursing station at Port Saunders, our planned destination, and we found we were not the only ones in trouble. The nursing station had a boiler breakdown and had been cold all day. Two maintenance men were driving from St. Anthony and were not expected until evening. Jo Hull, the eye nurse, was coming with them. We were advised to find accommodation on the way and to try to reach them the next day, when it was hoped heating would be re-established.

There was seal meat on the menu that evening, for seal is harvested by the inshore fishermen for food as well as pelts. I found it tasted like liver, and I enjoyed it. Seal flippers are considered a delicacy, as are cod tongues.

We made it to Port Saunders, then to Flower's Cove, but though there was no obvious radiator leak, the car problem continued until St. Anthony, where a defective pressure cap on the radiator was replaced, curing the problem. I was to learn a lot about being more prepared for emergencies on that trip, such as taking extra gasoline and a second shovel.

"Joey" did what he could to provide work for Newfound-landers. For example, *Strathcona III*, a new hospital ship, was built for the I.G.A. in the shipyard of Messrs. E. G. Barnes Ltd. in St. John's. I was to ride in this ship shortly after its launching in 1965. We were scheduled to do a clinic at a small community

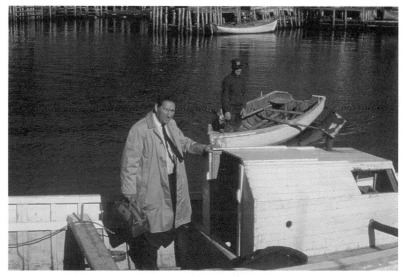

Captain Small of the Strathcona III with fisherman in an open dory.

of Grandois, and, as we were to leave at dawn, we slept aboard the ship. Captain Norman Small started at day-break, but once out of St. Anthony harbour, we found a side wind and chop on the sea at Hare Bay. The harbour entrance at Grandois is narrow, giving good protection for the small boats, but with a low tide, wind, and narrow entrance, the *Strathcona* had to be carefully edged in.

As we were being rowed ashore, we could see the smoke curling up from the schoolhouse, and, when we arrived, the blankets were up on the windows for blackout, so we could start immediately. The weather, being too rough for the small boats to go fishing that day, was a help to us, as it meant that if we found some inherited eye defect we could access both parents.

When our clinic was over, we were informed that the *Strathcona* was waiting for us at St. Julien's, the next cove down the coast. This had a more commodious entrance and was where the ships collecting the local catch of cod from the inshore fishermen often berthed. As it was still too rough for us to sail around the coast in a fishing boat, we crossed the hill that separated the two coves, walking single-file. The nurse, optician, and I each carried pieces of importance, while six of our young patients each carried a small item. The larger box, carefully roped, was carried suspended from an oar by two fishermen who volunteered. As our safari-like group crested the hill, we could see *Strathcona*'s trim lines in the cove. We were soon picked up by her lifeboat and sailing on to our next clinic at Conche.

On another trip to Conche, I entered in a much less conventional way, much to the amusement of the citizens. The phone jangled me awake on Sunday morning at 8:00 a.m. Dr. John Gray, who was Acting Administrator in Dr. Gordon Thomas's absence from the Grenfell Hospital at St. Anthony, Newfoundland, was on the line. There was a trip planned to visit Conche by the hospital ship, the *Strathcona*, but it was operating off the coast of Labrador and had not returned. So it was decided that we would go by plane on the Sunday afternoon, so we could start work on Monday morning.

The voice was saying: "The weather probs are bad for the afternoon, but flying is excellent now. How soon can you be ready, Graham?" I felt like saying "never," as I was looking forward to another hour of sleep. It had been a tiring week of work at Port Sauders followed by surgery at St. Anthony. Unfortunately, weather is king on the coast of Newfoundland, so I said, "10:30." I knew there was a lot to do: rouse the optician and secretary to go with me, pack the equipment, and see the patients in the wards, as I would not be back for three or four days.

We nearly made it! The plane was loaded for take-off on floats as the church bells started to call the people to church for the 11:00 a.m. service. We climbed up over the hospital and town, then headed south over the fishing hamlet of Goose Cove, and out over Hare Bay. We were to drop off a child returning to the little village of Croque, after paediatric care in St. Anthony. Croque has a very narrow entrance, and I watched with interest to see how the pilot would manage the descent. He touched down, then guided the plane down the harbour to see if the tide was high enough to allow the wing to clear. Finding it so, he turned the plane around so that the wing overlapped the wharf. By gently guiding the wing he was able to bring the plane in close enough so that the child could be handed into the arms of the people waiting for him.

A push on the wing from the shore and the touch of the throttle had the de Havilland Otter ready for take-off. The pilot, Tom Green, was talking to Miss Jo Catell (the nurse in charge at the Conche nursing station) on the radio as to where the best place was to land. We set down beside a small skiff anchored in the harbour as a marker. As all the people in Conche are devout Roman Catholics, only those who were to attend to our needs were around. A small boat with an outboard motor put out to meet us manned by a boy. We soon found that our equipment filled it and the boy would have to make another trip. In order to let the plane proceed to Gander before the "weather" came down, we decided to wait in the anchored skiff.

It seemed to have "sweated a bit," (a euphemism for water spilling about in it) and it looked very flimsy to me. The secretary, optician and I each descended in turn, walked along the float and entered the boat. At least the first two did. I did not think it could stand the sudden jar of my descent and so I tried to step into it gingerly. I had forgotten that both the float and boat were moveable and I did not have a firm base from which to step. I stepped too gingerly only to find one side entered the boat and the other did not. Thus the left leg and side was wet as the boat keeled over to forty-five degrees. The other two in the boat soon had it righted and strong arms pulled me aboard. As soon as I was safely in the skiff, the plane moved away.

I never was sure whether there was a chuckle from the plane's cockpit or whether it was the water lapping on the sides which I heard. The other two members of the party behaved with suitable poise and we were brought to the wharf by the boy in his little boat. As we tied up, a voice enquired as to who was the one who got wet. I had to confess that it was I. "In Englee they dip them every Sunday," came the reply. This was my introduction to Miss Jo Catell. She was, of course, referring to the fact that at Englee, further down the coast, the Pentecostal community was strong and baptism by immersion

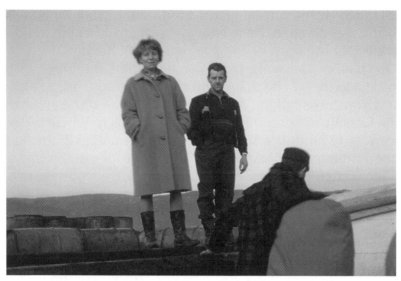

Jo Catell, waiting to receive a not quite all wet ophthalmologist.

was a frequent Sunday rite.

Soon I was in the nursing station and while my clothes dried, I was able to finish the "spot of horizontal" from which I had been roused in the morning. In the afternoon, after my clothes had dried sufficiently, we were able to take a walk around Conche. The island derives its name from its apparent resemblance on a map to a sea shell. One of the interesting features is the small house which acted as a nursing station during visits in Dr. Grenfell's time. Now the nursing station is well built and has beds for emergency care and obstetrics. It reflects the background of the nurse, Miss Catell, who was in the nursing section of the paratroop division during World War II. No officer's Sam Browne or buttons could shine brighter than the station's floors. There was no spit, but plenty of polish! This was preserved by the discipline maintained as all the fishermen were taught to remove their heavy boots and wear provided slippers when coming for treatment.

Next morning we opened our clinic in the auditorium attached to the school, using the curtains to close off the stage for the darkness required for eye examinations. Some treatments were carried out in the nursing station close at hand. One of these required the syringing of a blocked tear duct. I explained to the fisherman that if I were successful he would feel the saline in his throat.

"You would know how the salt feels in your throat, would-n't you, Doc!", he said with a grin.

As a matter of fact, I had not been so deeply immersed that I had had water in my throat, but I knew that the wave from my plunge had reached the shore. I felt sure that the boy had increased the tale to one taller than himself. In all probability I had been reported as going down for the third time until rescued by him and his sturdy little boat.

He seemed to enjoy the joke, so I laughed with him anyhow!

As a physician, Grenfell had always sought the deeper and interrelated causes of disease, which he had felt were the deep poverty and illiteracy of the people. The illiterate fisherman was at a disadvantage when bargaining for the price of his fish catch, and for the staples such as flour purchased from the trading vessels. This was one of the reasons for the formation of co-operatives, some of which still exist. Viable work schemes had also to be developed, but one which was to bring reindeer and Lapland herders failed. Others succeeded with the help of Dr. Curtis to carry them through: a farm, a dairy, a drydock for schooners, and cottage industries. These provided work and reduced dependence on imports.

Smallwood had similar problems. He needed a work force that was educated, but the budget for 1200 communities around the coast in 1933 was $509,138.[7] Obviously, many places had no teachers. In a sense, Smallwood was worse off than Dr. Grenfell had been, for as a Mission, he could ask for volunteers in the high schools and universities in the United States, Britain, and Canada, and they came to help. A government could not take this approach. To reduce the need to supply so many commun-ities with services of all kinds, such as electric light, roads, and schools, more isolated outports were brought into larger units. I saw this occurring when visiting the south coast in 1968: houses were being moved on barges, which in many cases, pro-duced considerable distress to those uprooted.

Like Grenfell, Smallwood had a wide vision of what was required to develop the resources of Newfoundland, but while he had made mistakes in office, which he frankly admits,[8] he also had successes. One of these in which I had a small share was the Churchill Falls project.

For many years, it had been known that Labrador not only held great riches in minerals, but also had a fabulous renewable resource—water for hydroelectric energy. This was because the plateau was saucer-shaped with Michikamau Lake in the centre, which was kept high by heavy snow and rainfall. The only release for this was by the Hamilton River, which fell through a five-mile stretch of rapids, then over the falls into the gorge below. It continued to descend through Bowdoin Canyon, so that fifteen miles below the falls, the difference of elevation from the plateau above had reached 1,060 feet. This provided a natural site for a hydroelectric power development of great magnitude. If this could be tapped, power could be sold to the United States at considerable profit. Sir Wilfred Grenfell records being awed by the falls' majesty and potential, as they were one and a half times the height of the falls at Niagara, when he accompanied an aerial survey being carried out by Alexander Forbes and Charles Hubbard in 1935.[9]

How could this rich resource be developed? There were two main obstacles. One was ownership of the land. Quebec laid claim to much of Labrador in 1902, and it took twenty-five years before the border was settled in Newfoundland's favour. There had been much acrimony, and the resulting bitterness would bedevil later negotiations. The other, as always, was money. An estimated five billion dollars was needed for the Upper Churchill Falls alone. Another scheme to tap the river further down at Gull Island Rapids and the Muskrat Falls to bring cheap power to Newfoundland's envisioned industry would require separate financing.

In spite of the enormous cost, the opportunity to create 30,000 jobs and bring millions of dollars annually into the treasury was worth the effort, and so Smallwood visited Sir Winston Churchill in London. With his help, a major syndicate called Brinco (headed by the British house of de Rothschild) was put together. To recognize his assistance, the name "Hamilton Falls" was changed to "Churchill Falls." (Unfortunately, another place called "Churchill," and a "Churchill River," already existed in Canada.)

The work force was so large, and the construction so dangerous—blasting 3,000,000 cubic yards of precambrian rock, and building eighty dykes—that the hospital was one of the first things constructed. It was natural, as the I.G.A. was operating medical facilities in Labrador already, that Dr. Gordon Thomas should be asked to staff the unit with a fully qualified general surgeon. Dr. John E. Price was chosen.

The dykes were to raise depressions in the edges of the spoon-like plateau so that a water basin, with half the capacity of Lake Ontario could be created—the third biggest man-made lake in the world, at that time. It was to be called "Smallwood Reservoir." The water was then to be guided through ten penstocks, cut out of the rock and lined with cement. The water would then fall on ten giant generators, two and a half times the power of any others in use. As the water returned to the river below the canyon, it dropped 1,000 feet onto the turbine blades.

My first visit to the falls was in 1967, when there were only bunk houses and a large common dining hall. A townsite was rapidly built with permanent housing, hotel and shopping mall. Wives and families of those who would stay permanently, or at least during the five years of construction, also required a school. My duties as a visiting consultant were mainly with this population, as many of the shorter-term construction workers had frequent leave and saw me only for infection or minor eye trauma.

It was not until my third visit to the area that I was able to see the falls themselves, as they were situated on the road to Esker, about fifteen miles from the townsite. I had been able to borrow a car, and found the well-worn track to a cairn with a plaque telling that the first white man to see this great sight was John McLean, who, in 1839, visited the district as a factor for the Hudson's Bay Company. The spray from the cataract dampened my clothes as it rose 200 yards to keep the sun's rays from melting the snow still lying near the edge. It was power just waiting to be converted to use!

It was easy for accidents to happen in an area with such construction activity, as the following case illustrates. When a construction worker was guiding a giant hydroelectric turbine being lowered by crane on a platform, the platform tipped slightly, throwing off the 300-pound man, who was also steadying the turbine. Unfortunately, as he fell, he also crushed the engineer, who was only half his weight. The engineer, badly bruised all over and with eyes swollen shut, was taken to the hospital. After the swelling subsided and he returned to work, he found visual field changes, as well as distortion of images. He was referred to me and was found to have a torn retina with progressing retinal detachments. He was quickly flown to Toronto, where the retinal surgeon, Michael Shea, was able to reattach the retinae. Fortunately, he was able to return to work and even to his hobby of painting. I have long ago lost touch with the man, but a picture I still retain of a sunset on Smallwood Reservoir reminds me of the episode.

I have long believed that the spirits of those who have gone before are cognisant of much that happens in the sphere they left. If this is true, then I believe that Sir Wilfred Grenfell's spirit must have looked down in satisfaction that this water resource was producing so much continued blessing. Twenty-one thousand Newfoundlanders were able to earn $121 million, while many Quebecois benefited similarly. One other benefit that would have given Grenfell great happiness is that over the crags and the valleys the great transmission lines carried electric power to the northern United States. During the years of distress in the northern peninsula and in Labrador, much money had been collected in that country, and many of its citizens had given time as "workers without pay" (or "WOPs")[10] and teachers. Now Labrador was yielding its resource to give them light and power. Newfoundland's government was also assured of $16 million annually, as long as the water flowed.

He would be particularly pleased that the virtual isolation of Labrador for over eight months of the year had been broken by the "short take-off and landing (STOL)" air ambulance, with pick-up from settlements to the hospitals. If this had been in place seventy-five years before, he would not have broken through the ice on Hare Bay and nearly died to reach a sick child.

I was to see many of these changes during the years 1964–76 in my visits to the northern peninsula and Labrador. The medical facilities of the new Harry L. Paddon Hospital at Happy Valley (named after one of Dr. Grenfell's early recruits) was opened in 1965. The new hospital for St. Anthony, Charles Curtis Memorial was not officially opened until 1968, but well before that time, the crowded quarters of the O.T. room in the old building were abandoned for generous space in the new. It was very gratifying to have room for instruments, and electric outlets where we needed them, for we had had input in the design.

Added to this was the fact that Miss U. J. Hull was seconded from her work as Public Health Nurse to co-ordinate the visits in the far-flung practice, and to see that those patients requiring mandatory recall were rechecked in those outports.

These extra facilities added much to the organising of the records and the family trees which we were forming. Dr. Gordon Johnson, who was to follow me in St. Anthony was able to develop the work further in his genetic and other studies.

While Newfoundlanders suffered from the same eye defects as others around the world, some were the product of local environment and geography. One such had just been described by Freedman[11] and called "Labrador keratopathy." This condition was brought to the attention of Dr. Freedman, a British ophthalmologist making a short-term visit to northern Labrador, by Dr. Tony Paddon,[12] son of Dr. H. L. Paddon and director of the northern region of the Grenfell services. One of the first people to be noted with this condition was a postman whose duty it was to travel from settlement to settlement in winter by dog team. He found his vision was becoming reduced. Examination revealed clouding of the cornea to be limited to the area between the lids. On elevating the upper lid, the cornea was as clear as the glass it is supposed to resemble.

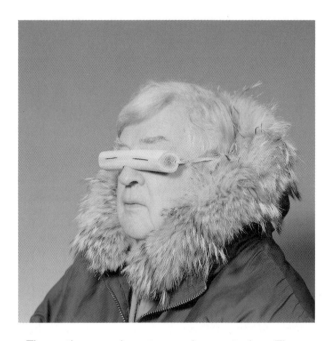

The author wearing stenopaeic spectacles. These lightweight spectacles are made from hollowed-out caribou antlers; the ties are of caribou hide. They protect the eyes from snowblindness and damage from ice crystals. Unlike sunglasses, they do not fog up. The use of stenopaeic slits dates back to the Thule people (800 to 900 years ago). The Inuit presumably learned it from them.

Dr. Freedman was aided in his description of the eye condition by the provision of a slit lamp, or biomicroscope, provided by the Canadian National Institute for the Blind (CNIB). This allowed Dr. Freedman to describe the condition accurately in the *Archives of Ophthalmology* in 1965. I was able to examine quite a few of these cases in my later visits, and confirm that they all had suffered from long exposure to the elements. My cases were in older males, most of whom gave a history of having been lost during blizzards. To prevent succumbing to the "sleep of death" during the blinding snow, they had kept their eyes open enough to move around. Besides ultraviolet light and snow blindness, during daylight hours, they were often exposed to fine spicules of ice which could pit the face as well as the eyes. One of the saddest cases I saw was that of a deaf mute, who was trapped in such a storm at night near his home. If he could have made himself heard above the storm, he might have been able to summon help.

The Inuit had solved the problem of eye protection years ago, by the use of ivory shields with slits which protected them from ice spicules as well as glare from harmful rays. Unfortunately, the white settler has often failed to appreciate the wisdom and experience acquired by natives, or to adopt his ways. For this he has often paid with disability or life itself. Prevention is the only effective method of dealing with the problem, but for one case

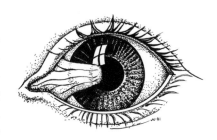

Pterygium.
(Sketch by Dr. J. Watt.)

with marked scarring I tried a corneal graft, using a partial thickness section of the patient's own cornea and rotating the clear portion from under the upper lid so that it lay over the pupil. While this improved the vision to some extent, the benefit was limited by the fact that the patient had an early cataract condition. No doubt my successor would have to remove the clouded lens when the vision was further reduced.

Another problem associated with the environment is the pterygium. In this condition there is a growth of the conjunctiva across the cornea. In most cases this is not severe enough to limit vision, but if allowed to grow it can involve the pupil area. It is a disease most often associated with hot, dry climatic conditions found in the Australian outback. In fact Pico[13] writing in the *World Congress of the Cornea*, states that this is a disease of the tropics and subtropics.

Having read this statement the evening before, I was forced to smile wryly when I found on my operating list—"removal of pterygium." It was snowing heavily outside and I found it hard to identify my car from the others parked below. I felt there must be another mechanism, as I could not compare these weather conditions with subtropics. In one random survey I found some signs of pterygium in thirty-three per cent of males over forty years of age. Most were fishermen or part-time lumbermen. I postulated that in the days of the open boat, the fisherman sailing into the rising sun was exposed to two doses of damaging sun rays—one direct and one reflected from the water. On the return trip he was often exposed to the same dosage from the setting orb. Not only did the eyes suffer but also the lower lip, which could have a form of cancer called fisherman's lip, similar to a condition described in the tropics by Nicolau and Bulus.[14] This condition was to disappear as fishermen learned that their lips could be protected by using some of their wife's lipstick. Later, the use of cabins changed the fishing boat so that sunglasses could be used without interference by spray of the water.

One thing still puzzled me. Why was pterygium fairly common on the northern peninsula, and rare in Labrador where keratopathy was more common? Unfortunately I have no exact statistics to bring to bear. We enquired about only the primary occupation, so if fishermen engaged in lumbering during the winter this would not appear on our records. The resins in sawdust are very irritable to the eye, and also there is potential hazard to the cornea from tree branches. Sometimes the conjunctiva could adhere to these injured areas producing a pseudo-pterygium.

There was much to investigate, but pressure of work and short stays precluded in-depth study. Now the conditions that produced some of the eye problems have gone. The slower dog team, with long exposure to sunglare, has been replaced except for sporting events by the rapid snowmobile with the rider protected by goggles. The open dory with oars has yielded, even for the in-shore fishermen, to the cabined motorised fishing boat. Greater education in prevention of hazards has also consolidated the gains made by technical progress.

But genetic traits are harder to alter, and in a close-knit society such as I found when I arrived in the Grenfell area, this determined much of the findings. Even up to the time of my last visit to the northern peninsula it was possible to guess what eye defects would be found by determining the name of the patient and the village from which he came. Patients coming from the community of Raleigh most often had high myopia. People with certain names probably had glaucoma or strabismus.

I was also to find similar "pockets" of genetic defects in isolated communities farther south such as Twillingate, New World Island and Fogo, where the greatest abnormalities of the iris of the eyes were seen.

Tuberculosis, which had been such a scourge on the coast in Sir Wilfred Grenfell's time, was brought under control by the vigilance and strenuous work of the early Mission doctors. By the time I visited the coast there was little evidence of the corneal problems I had found in Baffin Island. Dr. Tony Paddon tells how this was done in Volume V of *The Book of Newfoundland* under the title "Life in Labrador with my famous father."[15]

Dr. Harry Paddon, who like Grenfell often was skipper as well as physician, would take the seventy-five-foot ship *Maraval* into every inhabited cove and hamlet on the dangerous 300-mile strip of coast. More cautious than Grenfell, and as the coast was better charted, he never ran aground as Grenfell had.

After Dr. Harry's death in December 1939 his son Anthony, who had been born in Labrador, took over the work after his release from naval service in World War II. The *Maraval*, with new engine and X-ray equipment, was to serve the son as it had the father.

Meanwhile on the northern peninsula of the Island of Newfoundland similar efforts were being made with a tuberculosis sanitorium which opened in St. Anthony in 1953, replacing the thirty-bed annex which had been given by Mrs. Beatrice Fox Griffiths in 1937.

In spite of the war against it, tuberculosis was hard to eradicate—an unusual complication affecting the eyes of a child showed up in 1967. I had seen the seven-year-old child in 1965, when she had 20/30 vision. By 1967 she was having difficulty at school, with her right eye seeing 20/400 and the left counting fingers at one metre. There was a pale optic nerve, which suggested the presence of organic disease rather than hysteria, as can occur in the young. This was confirmed when Miss U. J.

Hull, who had previously been the public health nurse, recognized the name and remembered the child as having tuberculosis meningitis as a baby.

It so happened that I had recently attended an international conference in Montreal designed to coincide with the Man and His World exposition. There had been a lively discussion on damage to the optic nerves by adhesions formed after meningitis. The discussants had seen this more commonly in Europe than in North America. Could this be such a case? More investigation was needed, and so she was referred to Dr. R. J. Purvis, a paediatrician. Investigation revealed that adhesions had indeed blocked the circulation of the cerebro-spinal fluid. The dilated brain ventricles were pressing on nerves connecting the eye to the brain.

Dr. Gordon Thomas, who had previously trained with the famous neurosurgeon Dr. Wilder Penfield, was able to place a valve to allow the hydrocephalus to drain. This permitted the nerves to recover dramatically so that the vision returned to 20/30 with glasses, and facilitated her return to classes as an unhandicapped student. Cooperation such as this between nurses and specialists of different disciplines made our work in the North so successful.

This case was recorded in the *British Medical Journal*[16] and because of its rarity requests for reprints came to my office from North America, Europe and even from behind the Communist curtain.

Up until early 1968, I had been making trips from Toronto to the North or Grenfell zone and Central Newfoundland every three months, so I decided to take a leave of absence from September 1968 to September 1970. As I drove towards Port-aux-Basques, preparatory to making a move of some household effects, it was natural to remember some of the incidents of the past in the North. There had been much rewarding work, and there had also been an element of fun. There had been many firsts, especially in the outdoors.

I smiled as I remembered my first skidoo ride. Skidoos were not common when I first visited Mary's Harbour in 1964. There had been a blizzard and the plane had not been able to pick up the eye team. I had written a few letters but needed stamps. One young WOP (worker without pay) had learned to ride the new machine, and offered to take me to the store. The harbour we crossed was mostly bare from the strong wind, and we developed considerable speed before hitting a bank of snow, leaving a very frosty snowman to scramble out. Although it was obvious what had happened, the postmistress, like Newfoundlanders generally, was too polite to fuss over me, or comment about city slickers having their baptism in the white water of the northern winter.

I also thought of my first snowshoe trial and icefishing trip in Roddickton. As we had not been outdoors all week we decided to hold the clinic in the evening, and spend the day visiting a nearby lake where beautiful trout were being caught. To reach it we had to cross some deep snow, but fortunately our local guide had brought along snowshoes. I made it to the holes in the ice, marked by branches where others had fished. I was instructed by the optician, a Newfoundlander and keen outdoorsman. I had a bite and even got the trout to the hole. It was a big one, but I was not quick enough—with a sudden twist, he freed himself and was gone. Fortunately the optician had taken four beauties, so we snowshoed back. The sun had set just enough to illuminate the snow at an angle that brought out the purest blue from the crevices. The afternoon exercise gave extra taste to the fresh fish for supper, which I still remember.

It had been exciting to return to Toronto, which had been my home for twenty years, but a bigger challenge would await me as I returned to form a base in Grand Falls.

4 / *Move to Central Newfoundland*

Recognized rights of Canadians to full enjoyment of efficient vision.

Canadian Ophthalmological Society
statement of purpose and principle

M Y DECISION IN 1968 to take two years' leave of absence from my practice in Toronto evolved after considerable thought and was prompted by a number of factors.

The first was the apparent need. I had already been challenged as a doctor and as a Christian to provide care for those in Maritime outports. After the first trip I wrote to Dr. Millar, deputy minister of health in St. John's, and when he was in Toronto we met for lunch. He pointed out that what I had perceived as need in the northern peninsula of Newfoundland and in Labrador reflected the reality in central Newfoundland as well. There were only three ophthalmologists in St. John's and one in Corner Brook, 500 miles away. After our lunch I decided to try to schedule a trip to Newfoundland every three months, endeavouring to serve in the central and Grenfell areas.

On a visit to St. John's in 1967 I had gone with Dr. Millar to the Newfoundland headquarters of the Canadian National Institute for the Blind, on whose board he served. A need had been expressed by the public health nurse, who did routine eye examinations in schools in Gander and had found children with lazy eye with or without turn. When she rechecked months later the same children showed up, without having gone for treatment.

To have an eye examination and receive treatment in central Newfoundland was a matter of some economic concern, as it meant a trip to the capital, St. John's. Appointments took considerable time to obtain and usually required an overnight stay—seeing first the ophthalmologist, then the optician and afterwards the return trip. As there was no medicare prior to 1966, some people felt they could not afford the time or the expense. This was particularly true in the case of amblyopia—or lazy eye—diagnosed at school and usually advanced too far to bring back adequate vision. People with more than one child with this condition would complain to the nurse that they had already taken time and spent good money to get help without benefit, so why do it all again?

Now, if I could find a locum who would hold my practice together and cover expenses in Toronto, I could take two years' leave to work in Grand Falls on the eye problems of central Newfoundland. Such a specialist became available in Dr. Glazier Somerville, who had been in family practice in New Brunswick and was completing his work in the eye training course at the University of Toronto. (As it happened, he stayed in Toronto after my return and later became head of the ophthalmology department in North York Branson Hospital.)

One more question remained. As one who had been born of missionary parents, and who had received medical training through bursaries and grants, I had always felt that medicine was a sacred trust. Moreover, the Bible had always been my guide and compass—what did it say? The answer came in the First Epistle of John, 4. 17,18: "If anyone has material possessions and sees his brother has need but has no pity on him, how can the love of God be in him? Dear children, let us not love with words, but with actions and in truth." Like Wilfred Grenfell, who seventy-five years before had faced the challenge to help the needy, I too, if I wished to be called a Christian, had to put deeds before words. I could not offer anything but expertise, but this was what was needed.

So it was that I left my practice in the hands of Dr. Somerville and, with station wagon and trailer loaded with diagnostic and personal effects, left Toronto. I reached Ottawa about noon, had lunch with a dear friend, and said adieu.

The Trans-Canada Highway took me through Quebec, New Brunswick and Nova Scotia. It was fall, and the changing colours in these well-wooded provinces formed a plaid to warm the heart of a Scot like me. The crossing by ferry from Sydney,

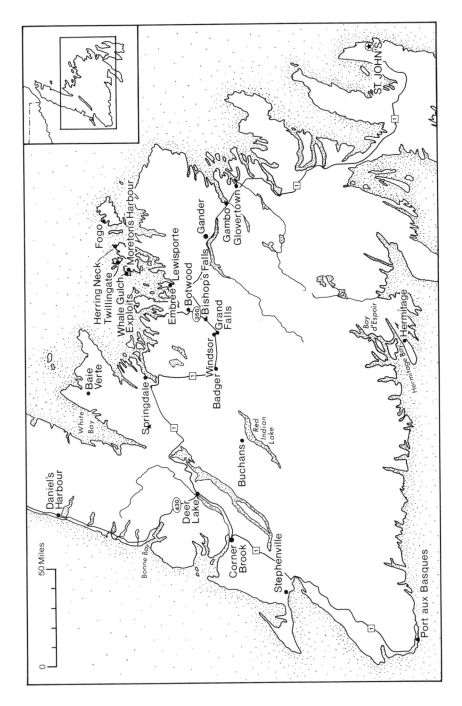

Central Newfoundland.

Nova Scotia to Port-aux-Basques, Newfoundland was fortunately not as rough as it sometimes is. I stayed near Corner Brook. Looking down on the city from the highway, it was impossible to miss seeing the haze which lay over the town below from the large Bowaters paper mill, which formed the economic heart of the community. Next morning I pushed on to Grand Falls, another paper-making town situated halfway across the island. For the next two years, with the atmospheric inversion so common in the mornings, I lived with the sulphur haze of the mill.

The road from Corner Brook was well paved. It was easy to make good time, as there was only one significant community at Deer Lake, where there is an airport and where the road to the northern peninsula turns off. I had travelled this section in 1965 when the 575-mile Trans-Canada was still under construction. Joey Smallwood was proud to be the last of the Fathers of Confederation when he spearheaded the union of Newfoundland with Canada on March 31, 1949. He was still the province's Liberal premier and was never hesitant to proclaim that the benefits which Newfoundland enjoyed were due to his close relationship with the Liberal government in Ottawa. Along the highway there had been signs: "We'll finish this drive in '65 thanks to Lester Pearson."

I had arranged to have an apartment and an office at the Medical Arts Building close to the Central Newfoundland Hospital in Grand Falls. I arrived early enough to unpack that day, and after about a week had the office in operation.

Grand Falls, which was to be my base for the next two years, was a planned community—unlike most of the coastal outports in Newfoundland. Grand Falls had been chosen in order to develop water power generated by the falls on the Exploits River, and also because of the abundant wood in the area. The Anglo-Newfoundland Company had obtained a ninety-nine-year lease and built a pulp mill in 1909. Around the mill the company town grew until 1961, when the mill was purchased by the Price brothers and the town became a self-governing municipality with its own mayor.

While the town was under company control, non-essential services desired by the population started springing up on the opposite side of the railway tracks where a community called Grand Falls Station developed. The growth of this area was not organized until 1942, when it became the town of Windsor. By 1968, the two centres had a combined population of about 14,000.

Before long my professional office in Grand Falls became too small, so I obtained a house near the centre of the city on Hill Road. I was able to live on the upper floor and had the commodious lower area for a waiting room. As many of the patients came from small, remote communities, I was able to hire an optician to fit the glasses I prescribed, and so save the patient a second trip.

Surgery was conducted at the Central Newfoundland Hospital in Grand Falls and the James Paton Memorial Hospital in Gander. To this latter hospital I travelled twice a week, and the days were long. I would see patients in Grand Falls before breakfast, then drive sixty miles to Gander. As there was only one traffic light between the two hospitals it was usually possible to travel the distance in an hour, if there were no hazards. Incredibly, although the winter snow was heavy with drifts on each side higher than the average car, there were only two occasions in two years in which the Royal Canadian Mounted Police had to close the highway, forcing me to cancel my clinic.

Gander, with a population of 10,000, was a town surrounding an airport. Until the arrival of high-flying jets with greater fuel capacity, Gander was a staging and refuelling base on trans-Atlantic flights. I had visited the airport in 1950 when travelling to see my mother shortly before she died, but at that time I had no indication its streets—named after prominent flyers such as Amelia Earhart—would become well-known to me. When I had visited St. Anthony in 1964, the Gander hospital was new. It was to do yeoman service when a Cubana Airlines plane crashed at the end of the runway. As nearly all the people in Gander were in some way associated with flying, there was no need to call for volunteers—they came in droves.

The hospital received a citation from the Cuban government for its care of the burn victims, all of whom survived.

Usually I reached Gander by 9:30 a.m. and saw patients scheduled for surgery that day, and those I had operated upon on the last visit. The post-operative hospital stay was longer than in large cities, where follow-up is easy and frequent. Surgery would be conducted later in the morning and after lunch there was the out-patient clinic, where those from remote outports were waiting. Sometimes those from island communities would find it impossible to return home the same day, but many had relatives with whom they could stay. After supper I visited those operated upon that day, followed by the drive back to Grand Falls. Return trips were usually slower, especially if it had been snowing all day and the snowplows were on the road. Then the trip might be two hours, and I would arrive home between 10 p.m. and midnight.

As I was the only ophthalmologist between St. John's and Corner Brook, patients visited Grand Falls from as far north as Herring Neck on New World Island. While the distance ws not great by mainland standards, the weather and ferry services could make for an arduous journey. There was no causeway to Twillingate at that time, so a ferry carried people across the gap. On the one occasion in which I made this trip, the spring break-up was occurring. The wind changed direction and the crossing filled with icepans. The large ferry was out of commission but a smaller ferry was operating. It tried to weave between icepans, but sometimes the bow would rise alarmingly up on one. Then the ferry would pull back to shake it off, and try another passage. By the time I returned, however, the wind had pushed the ice seaward, and I had a clear passage back to the mainland and Grand Falls.

From the south, patients came from the areas around Bay d'Espoir and Hermitage Bay. On one interesting week I was able to accompany Mr. M. J. Colford, field secretary of the CNIB for central Newfoundland, on a five-day boat trip to see some of his blind clients from St. Albans—some as far away as François on the south coast. It was a holiday from eye work, but invaluable from an educational point of view. Fishermen and fish plant workers toiled in little communities where houses clung like limpets to rocky cliff faces. How the blind coped with paths where there were no flat areas, where each step was either up or down, was remarkable. The coast was so rugged that the sea was their only highway.

Patients also came from the southeast—from Buchans, near Red Indian Lake, where the Beothuks had made their last desperate stand. They came too from Springdale, and Badger on the Trans-Canada Highway. I also held clinics at Baie Verte, where the United Church had a hospital.

History has always had a fascination for me, and so on one of my quarterly trips to St. Anthony I was talking with one of the staff physicians about the new finds in the northern tip of the peninsula, at L'Anse aux Meadows. As he had his car it was decided that just after church his wife would make a picnic lunch, and we would drive north to look over the site. Although we had no guide and the ruins were still being excavated, it was easy to imagine the story of the Norsemen as I looked across the sward at L'Anse aux Meadows.

It had been known for a long time that the Vikings came into the area of the straits when Liev the Lucky Eiriksson sailed from Greenland across the Davis Strait to Baffin Island, which he called Helluland, or Land of Flat Stones. Then he turned south to skim the coast of Labrador, which he called Markland because it was wooded. Sailing south once more, he arrived at Vinland, but the position of that remained a mystery until Helge Instad discovered the site at L'Anse aux Meadows.

Before him, researchers and archeologists searching for Vinland down the coast from New England to Florida had been hoping to find an area where wild grapes grew. Helge, interpreting "Vin" by its early Norse meaning of "grass," realized he was looking for a meadow, not a vineyard, and tried Newfoundland. While at the Grenfell Mission headquarters at St. Anthony, he heard from a fisherman named George Decker, who suggested, "You might try Lancey Meadows. They say there are ruins hidden in the grass near Black Duck Creek."

Sure enough this was the answer, for the next year an expedition led by Helge and his archaeologist wife, Anne Stine

Ingstad, were able to uncover ruins of a typical Norse longhouse. More confirmatory evidence came to light at the diggings at L'Anse aux Meadows. A smithy was located where crude iron pyrites found nearby had been converted to bog iron for repair of tools or making nails for shop repairs.

Two small items were found which were of extreme importance to the team of archaeologists—the first was a bronze ring-headed pin, used by Vikings to fasten their cloak on the right shoulder, thereby freeing their arm for wielding a sword. The second was a spindle whorl, used by the Norse women to make yarn from wool.

Liev the Lucky built a house and stayed a year. His brother Thorvald came with intent to stay, but during further exploration he met natives with whom he fought, and by whom he was killed. That expedition returned to Greenland after two years.

Now as I dream, I can see the mist rising from the sea, leaving a heavy dew on the grass. I can imagine three ships offshore, like giant leviathans with dragon-like carved-wood prows and low, square woollen sails. In the prow of the leading vessel is Torfinn Karlsefni. He looks across and sees the house that Liev has built. This is indeed the area to which he had planned to bring his sixty men, five women and domestic animals to form a new colony.[1]

Running the ship into the entrance of Black Duck Creek, Torfinn jumps into the water and wades ashore. Six of his men follow, and with helmets gleaming in the rising sun they march on either side of their leader to Liev's old house. Finding it uninhabited and in reasonable repair, Torfinn raises his drawn sword to signal a general landing.

Gudrid, Torfinn's wife, is glad to wade ashore. Although this had not been a long trip as Viking journeys went, for Liev's landmarks had been found easily, she is pregnant and the added pitching of the vessel had reduced her tolerance for the stored food. She lies face down upon the field, rejoicing at the dew on her face and her tongue. She feels little Snorri's hands and feet beating in her womb, as if he too is happy for the landfall, and with some prescience she knows he will be the first of many of European stock to be born in this new land.[2]

I am called from my reverie by my guide pointing to the fire pits. How many great feasts had been prepared there? On the night of their arrival two sheep from their flock had been sacrificed, and Gudrid had claimed the skin as a resting place for her expected son. The wool would be spun by his mother for covering. Did she drop the spindle whorl which was to be found over 900 years later?

In spite of the optimism with which the colony was founded, it lasted only six years. It has been suggested that pressure from the native Beothuks brought this about, but the Norse were not known to back down from any fight. It seems much more plausible that the colony, deceived by the appearance of grass at the original site, might have thought the rest of the island was like this, only to discover muskeg and rock. The farms on Greenland must have looked more prosperous and inviting. Unless more women were brought into the colony, the disproportion of males to females could lead to a breakdown of the social structure. Whatever occurred, by about 1024 the Vikings had gone and the red-ochred Beothuk had the island to themselves.

Abandoning my reverie, we returned home from the picnic to our own more immediate problems. The delivery of effective medical care in Newfoundland and Labrador has always been bedevilled by the three main problems of scattered population, poor communication (especially in the winter months) and the poor economic base.

Around the larger communities, such as Grand Falls and Corner Brook with their pulpmills, and Gander with its international airport, employees had access to prepaid health plans. Residents of fishing villages and lumbering camps, however, were cared for under a cottage hospital scheme which the government tried to run from a minimum tax base. Even with a lower fee-for-service schedule than the mainland and the use of hospital-based salaried physicians, budgeted funds dried up before the new financial year began in April. One paediatrician in Grand Falls told me he regularly had to borrow around Christmas. The banks were willing to lend, knowing the money coming after the passing of the new budget in April would retire the debt.

Since the union of Newfoundland and Canada in 1949, there had been no shortage of immigrant medical personnel, many well-qualified, whose skills were not accepted in other provinces because of language or bureaucratic difficulties, but who could come to Newfoundland. There, with the help of colleagues, they could prepare themselves to take examinations set by the Medical Council of Canada. I had taken these licentiate examinations myself in Winnipeg, in 1948, although I had not the burden of learning another language.

Another benefit Newfoundland derived from Confederation, from an ophthalmologist's point of view, was the linkage of low-vision and blind people on the island with the facilities of the Canadian National Institute for the Blind (CNIB).

The story of this organization illustrates that God's providence can bring good out of man's greatest stupidity—war. In 1916, a sniper's bullet destroyed both eyes of Lt. E. A. Baker. After a period in St. Dunstan's in London, England, where many blinded residents of the United Kingdom were rehabilitated, Baker returned to his native Canada where he earned his living as a dictaphone typist for Ontario Hydro, transcribing trouble reports received by telephone.

Both Baker and A. G. Viets, the first Canadian soldier blinded in World War I, knew Canada was not prepared for later casualties. Knowledge of Baker's ability to organize must have reached high places, for he was promoted to colonel by the federal government and given the task of training and caring for the war-blinded.

Intercommunication and education of the blind had been made possible by Louis Braille, who in 1829 used a system of six dots to form an alphabet. This had become internationally accepted, and by 1907 enough books had been collected in Canada to form a lending library in Toronto. Distribution was aided by the federal government, which granted free mailing of braille material in 1898. Sharing the library space in Toronto, the Canadian National Institute for the Blind was formed on March 30, 1918.

The task given the founders was enormous, as the work soon expanded to cover civilians. There existed no standards as to what degree of visual impairment constituted industrial blindness, nor how many people across the country required the services offered. A registry had to be created of those blinded by disease as well as by trauma. As so much of this latter group consisted of workers blinded unnecessarily, prevention became a major plank in the program.

It was not until the early 1950s that I met Col. Baker. He made a habit of visiting the Canadian Ophthalmological Society meetings annually, and insisted on meeting the "newcomers" who would be caring for some of his "flock." I was impressed with his slim build and evident energy, but most of all with his "vision" of the potential of blind workers.

Because of the vastness of the country, provincial CNIB centres were formed and local employment opportunities developed. At first, jobs were rather menial—such as brush- and basket-making—but as experience and technology developed and the education level of the blind increased through braille and visual aids, openings were created in scholastic and technical fields. Some workers in Newfoundland were themselves products of CNIB training, and were in turn able to help others. Such a one was Eugene Pike, who with the assistance of the CNIB earned a Bachelor of Arts degree at Memorial University; he has now recently returned as Executive Director of the CNIB in Newfoundland.

In the remote areas of Newfoundland there was always a dread that failure of the specialized equipment used in ophthalmology would make our work difficult or impossible. Fortunately, as I am no mechanic, the engineers in charge of maintenance in the hospitals in Newfoundland were familiar with the necessity of ready adaptation. They never let me down.

In Gander, I had trouble with the electric motor of an erisophake (a suction apparatus used for the removal of cataracts). I had heard from a friend of an electrical company in town so I took it there to identify the trouble. I was told the best man in town for electric motors was Mr. H. Crewe, the chief engineer in the hospital. Sure enough, he kept it going through my stay in Newfoundland.

Similarly, in Grand Falls a lensometer (for measuring the prescription of patients' glasses) was damaged in transit and the bulb was broken. Neither Mr. Bennett, the chief engineer, nor I, had ever seen the inside of one of these instruments. To add to our trouble, I had no spare bulb available. While I returned to my clinic Mr. Bennett worked on the instrument. In a short time he returned; the instrument was working once more, a Christmas light bulb producing the illumination.

While conducting clinics at the M. J. Boylen Hospital in Baie Verte, a switch on the projectochart ceased to function. As it could not be fixed in the hospital itself, the help of the engineers at the Advocate Mines was sought. They found a car switch which fitted so well that it was still being used one year later.

A similar story could be told about St. Anthony. Junior Mesher had a natural capacity for understanding the complexity of medical instruments. One instrument which operated by remote control gave trouble. As it was still under warranty, I suggested it be sent back to the distributor. When it was returned it was still not working properly and was handed over to Junior, who found two wires were transposed.

Sometimes extemporization had to be carried out without expert assistance. This was necessary when visiting nursing stations—particularly in winter when bulbs were apt to blow if transported any distance in the cold and then used too soon. On one occasion it was necessary to borrow a bulb from a deep freezer to keep an instrument working.

Sometimes the most useful gadgets for extemporary repairs and general usefulness were clothes pegs and tie clips. On several occasions, I had difficulty with the automatic choke on my car. This would happen at the most awkward times, such as when I had been called to the Central Newfoundland Hospital late one evening. It was about midnight on a Saturday when I left to drive home. All the service stations were closed and most of the town was dark. The car stalled and would not start.

Sure enough, the choke had stuck. Opening it was easy—but how to keep it open while I started the car? By slipping a tie clip on the side of the carburettor to keep the butterfly valve open, it was possible to keep the car running. Once running, the clip was removed and the air filter replaced. After this I kept a clothes peg handy in the car. Beside its conventional purpose it was used to keep papers and charts together, and as I was given to having nosebleeds frequently and a colleague had informed me that the nares should be compressed for five minutes by the clock, the application of a clip saved a lot of time. The hands could be kept busy while the haemostat did its work. Surely the person who invented the spring clip must rank close behind the inventor of the wheel.

The sea has always been an integral part of the life of the Newfoundlander. It can be rough and cruel but it can also be beautiful and calm. On one lovely day I launched a small twelve-foot cartop aluminum boat on Lewisporte harbour and, with a friend who knew the way, travelled round the coast to Embree. Here we made a tour of the lobster traps which my friend had set. I had been particularly anxious to see how this work, which formed a significant part of Newfoundland's economy, was conducted.

Finally we tied up the little boat at the government dock among considerably larger fishing boats. Some people on the dock, looking down as the five-horsepower outboard edged up, asked where we had come from.

"From Lewisporte," we said.

"In that?"

It was true it had been a fun trip, but the boat was much more suitable for the rivers and inland lakes of Ontario from which I had brought it.

While there was much routine ophthalmology, there were also special challenges in genetic problems such as nystagmus (or "dancing eyes")and preventive ophthalmology associated with the early detection of lazy eyes, or amblyopia.

The trail of the dancing eyes started in February 1969 with what seemed to be a routine referral letter from Dr. John Sheldon in New World Island. The patient obviously had some difficulty seeing and he had nystagmus, which was easy enough to see as he handed me the note. The letter had a second page on which the doctor's nurse, a local girl, had traced a family tree indicating that the boy the patient had brought with him, and who had the same last name, had the same condition and was also his nephew. I did not realize it at the time, but this letter was the start of a project involving months of investigation, which included three ophthalmologists, the CNIB, miles of road travel and even visits by water to coastal islands where some of the 200 people involved lived.

The two patients could only be corrected to 20/200 (the large letter on the test chart) and were therefore candidates for registration with the CNIB. To my dismay, that same week a mother brought two small children into the hospital in Gander with almost exactly the same features of the previous cases. Although they came from an area about 100 miles from the first pair, the mother acknowledged that there was a distant relationship.

It seemed there was going to be a great expenditure of time and travel if the origin of this problem was to be unravelled. As I was operating alone in central Newfoundland, with a session every three months in St. Anthony and the Grenfell area, I felt I could not spare the time. I therefore wrote to my friend Dr. Gordon Johnson,[3] who was in his research year of a fellowship in ophthalmology in Toronto, explaining the problem and asking if he could take time off to help with the investigation. He could. As the cases were to come under the supervision of Mr. Colford,[4] the CNIB representative for central Newfoundland, I also sought his help. We were able to extract from CNIB files the names of those who were already registered with nystagmus, and some of those fitted into the family tree, which seemed to have two branches, one in the New World Island area and one in the Badger area.

By the time Dr. Johnson arrived, more cases had been identified and with the help of Mr. Colford and CNIB transportation, the first visits were planned. We felt there must be a link between the two branches, and Dr. Johnson found it in New World Island. With some difficulty, he was able to interview a very elderly resident who, although intensely deaf, was made to understand the purpose of the visit. There, sitting on a bag of peas in the back of a store with charts spread before him, the old man was able to identify people who had married so the branches of the tree became one trunk. The chase took him back through six generations and 130 years to a lady who had carried the gene of ocular albinism from the south of England, married, and settled in the area of Moreton's Harbour or Whale Gulch, New World Island.

In this study, thirty-five males were discovered with "dancing eyes," and twenty-nine of these were examined.[5] The other six were working either in some remote island fishing or lumbering on the Canadian mainland. Unfortunately nothing therapeutic could be offered, but most of these men had learned to cope with their disabilities. Although not able to drive, most of them had been able to earn their living in the local setting, especially after visual correction with glasses. Although the skin pigmentation was normal, the appearance of the retina was that of an albino. The patients also had rather diaphanous irises and so a major complaint was that of photophobia, requiring strongly tinted glasses.

For these reasons the males tended to stay fairly close to their siblings, probably accounting for the fact that they had not scattered to the mainland like many other Newfoundlanders. They were also able to work by careful selection of jobs, in which the CNIB was able to assist. But even before the CNIB came into being, one of the first men afflicted with dancing eyes had been reputed to produce the best schooners in the district. He would check the planking with his hand and the finish by close inspection at a three-inch distance.

As the only help which could be given the male victims of this sex-linked condition was optical, it was in the females that we saw a glimmer of light. Was there some way in which we could distinguish the woman carrying the gene from her normal sister? This study was facilitated by the arrival of Dr. W. G. Pearce,[6] who was at that time based in Toronto. He had formerly studied genetics in Britain, and as well was an ophthalmologist. On his visit we were able to compare the distribution of retinal pigment in the unaffected and in the carrier. Blood samples were also taken for genetic analysis. It soon became clear that the unaffected female had full, even distribution of retinal pigment, while the sister who carried the abnormal gene showed patchy distribution, or streaks of pigment on a paler retina, as if painted with a drying brush.

Thus, being able to differentiate the two, we felt it was important that the female carrier know her options. For that reason, the full pedigree, with names, was left at CNIB headquarters in St. John's and in Toronto. Counselling by the ophthalmologist (who could read the signs in the eye), combined with birth control, seems the only obvious way to eradicate the abnormality.

One of the dreads of all health givers is patients who arrive too late for effective reversal of their problem. This is most common in ophthalmology with amblyopia, or lazy eye blindness. Sometimes amblyopia is discovered when children's eyes are examined at school. But this is often too late, as by the time children are in school it may be virtually impossible to persuade them to use or maintain occlusion of the good eye long enough to produce a return of adequate vision in the lazy eye.

In most cases, the best method of prevention lies in education. In the 1960s work was starting on ways of doing mass screening of the preschool population. Drs. S. B. Fainstein[7] and Ellis Shenken in Toronto were pioneers in the use of the Scarborough Screener. Dr. Shenken was also instrumental in obtaining a mobile van given by the Weston Lions Club for use as a base for eye service in small communities.[8] Because access was difficult in the northern peninsula and Labrador, children three-and-a-half to seven years old were screened during routine visits of the eye team from St. Anthony.

Alison Sayers coordinated these visits, which provided service to seventy-four communities on the mainland as well as to Labrador City and Wabush. In each of the areas, Miss Sayers sought the aid of volunteers and taught them the use of the Scarborough Screener. Of the 9,730 subjects screened, 1,389 failed and were referred to the nearest ophthalmologist for examination and follow up.

I was involved in surveys in Gander in October 1968, Grand Falls in February 1969 and Baie Verte in 1970, as well as a survey in the Grenfell area.[9] The amblyopia surveys were discontinued in 1971, when a mobile Eye Care Unit was set up. Alison Sayers left Newfoundland in 1973 and began lecturing in public health nursing at Queen's University in Kingston, Ontario.

Before I left Newfoundland in 1970, the government realized the arrival of medicare had increased the number of cases in the area, and recruited Dr. Mohdale Asgar, trained in ophthalmology in his native Pakistan, to take over the work based in Gander. We worked in close co-operation.

With the arrival of Dr. Asgar on July 1, 1969, the work based at the Gander Hospital was dropped from my shoulders. This allowed me to press on with other projects. I was soon in need of Dr. Asgar's surgical assistance, however, as a lady presented herself with a cataract in one eye and a corneal scar in the other which seemed amenable to corneal grafting. I had performed this surgery in Toronto, and had brought the trephines and other necessary instruments. The CNIB in Toronto operated an eye bank under Mrs. Ann Wolff, with whom I had communicated on several previous occasions.

Alerted of the need, Mrs. Wolff promised to telephone when suitable donor material was available. The patient, who lived in an outport, was brought to the hospital in Grand Falls for medical assessment and preparation. Two days later the telephone rang. An eye could be sent by Air Canada arriving at 11 p.m. Would I meet the flight in Gander? I would. In those days fresh tissue was shipped in special cooled containers, and the effective time for use was relatively short. I alerted the operating room staff and prepared my instruments for night surgery.

I saw the plane come in and raced to the agent. There was no shipment from the CNIB. The plane's steps were still down, so we hurried out to the tarmac just as its engines were starting. Did the stewardess have a special parcel?

"I'm so sorry; I was told to deliver this in Gander but I forgot," she confessed. It had been a close shave, for although the plane would return the next morning, so much time would have been lost that the chance of success would have been greatly reduced.

I had asked Dr. Asgar to work with me on the transplant. The graft was performed without a hitch, and as the lens behind the opacity was cataractous we removed it at the same time.

The next morning, on arrival at the hospital, I had a message to see the administrator. He wanted to know what had happened the night before. The news media had heard this was the first operation of its kind in Newfoundland and wanted a statement. The local radio station paid for tips on news items so the lady in the next bed, as we discovered later, slipped out to the telephone and rang her story in.

Corneal grafting was performed with much cruder material in those days. The finest suture material then available was 8 × 0 suture. Now 10 × 0 suture is used, requiring an operating microscope for placement and removal. Nevertheless, in spite of the donor material having travelled from Toronto to Gander by milk-run turboprop plane, followed by the sixty-mile drive to Grand Falls, there was no rejection. The patient was attended to by Dr. Asgar when I left the island the next year.

The facilities of the main office of the CNIB were always available, but the work and knowledge of the provincial organization made many worthwhile local projects possible.

A letter dated September 1990 from Mr. Eugene Pike, executive director of the CNIB in Newfoundland, informed me that Dr. Asgar is still working in Gander, and that he has been joined by three other ophthalmologists in covering central Newfoundland.

Meanwhile Miss U. J. Hull of the Grenfell Mission continued her work as the eye coordinator. In this capacity, she was able to arrange orderly coverage of the areas of greatest need on the long coastline serviced by the Grenfell Mission. She also kept lists of the cases of pathology for surgical intervention or review.

Jo, as most people knew her, spontaneously organized a map showing the occurrence of certain familial diseases, and by searching through the siblings we were able to identify those at high risk. Meanwhile, she could reach me in Grand Falls by telephone should any problem arise. Neither of us knew it then, but we were making a plan which I would later use in the Northwest Territories when starting the school of ophthalmic assistants in Yellowknife ten years later.

One of the things which kept Miss Hull busy while I was in central Newfoundland was the formation of family trees of glaucoma patients. Siblings of known glaucoma patients were plotted on a large wall map, and placed on recall lists in an effort to catch this disease in the early, treatable stage.

This effort at preventive ophthalmology could produce surprises. We found the administrator of the Grenfell Hospital at North West River was on the direct genealogical line of one such family. His condition was carefully monitored whenever we made a visit to that part of Labrador. The patient would otherwise have been missed as he had no symptoms, but as glaucoma is often called "the stealer by night," it is not unusual to have the condition found by routine check.

There could be social and international, as well as medical, surprises in Grand Falls too. One of these was the sudden appearance of President Kosygin of the Soviet Union into our midst one summer day.

The cold war between the U.S. and U.S.S.R. was at its height in June 1967, when on a clinical visit to Grand Falls, Newfoundland, the town became agog with the news that the Soviet leader Kosygin was arriving. I remember wishing that he was bringing his reported chill with him. I had left the heat and mugginess of Toronto behind as I thought, only to find that central Newfoundland was in the grip of a heat spell with the temperature rising to the 90's Fahrenheit. Not being equipped for such hot weather, there was no air conditioning in the hospital clinic—but I had been taken the day before to a natural pool for a cool-off swim. To reach this there was a short drive west on the Trans-Canada Highway to a club called Oasis. Parking there, a rough trail led upward beside Leech's Brook, over tree roots and boulders to the lower falls. Even further up was a deeper pool for the skilled swimmer. The water was warmer too, as to reach it the stream ran shallowly over a stretch of sun-soaked rock. Only in a place like Newfoundland where so much beauty is left unspoiled could one find a place like this without paved paths, chain-linked fence, and entry charge.

I was trying to keep cool by thinking of the evening dip when I heard the news. Premier Smallwood had received a message that Kosygin, who had been visiting Castro, was coming to Gander by a Cubana plane, which had regular refuelling privileges at that airport. Three choices were being offered him—a visit to St. John's, a fishing trip, or visit to the Price (Nfld.) Pulp and Paper Company in Grand Falls which was installing new equipment. This "whale of a machine," as Smallwood called it, was later to be named "Moby Joe." Kosygin, an engineer by profession, chose the latter. Fortunately a previous call to Mr. L. D. Wickwire, chief executive of the firm had warned him of this possibility, so allowed him to prepare a reception and light meal at the Grand Falls House. The lobster season had closed the day before, but thirty-eight fresh specimens were located in a local hotel.

The V.I.P. convoy consisting of Premier Smallwood, Kosygin, the Soviet Ambassador to Canada, the Second Secretary of the Soviet Embassy as interpreter, and the mayors of Gander and Grand Falls, soon devoured the sixty miles that separated the two towns. The Russian chief executive was in good form. He inspected the plant, talked to workmen, and even had a short walk about. The free enterprise stores were ignored as capitalistic but the main Co-op was considered as suitable to visit.

There was, of course, no pretence at secrecy in places the size of Grand Falls and Gander, but the most surprised person probably was the baby whose hand Kosygin shook during his visit to the Co-op store.

The trees at Grand Falls House provided a cooler place for refreshment and chat. The Soviet Ambassador enjoyed himself so much that he suggested that they should meet in Russia and see the paper mills there. But the Soviet Premier would have none of this "Comrade" stuff, he was still boss and rebuked the ambassador: "It is for me to invite, and for you to make the arrangements."[10]

The visit was soon over, as there was to be a meeting with De Gaulle in France in the morning, and Kosygin had to have a good sleep. The visit was cordial, and it was evident that "refrigeration" was only used when rival U.S. delegations were encountered.

I had not finished in time to see the participants, so as there had been no recorded change in the atmospheric conditions, the open invitation to the Leech's Brook was gladly accepted.

In September 1970, I had promised to return to my practice in Toronto. There was no ophthalmologist available to take over the practice at that time, though, after I left, one did come from the United States, so I had to rent my residence on Hill Road in Grand Falls and turn my vehicle westward.

Willowdale and I had both changed in the two years during which I had been on my leave of absence. Fortunately, the Northwestern, Branson, and North York General Hospitals had all kept my staff appointments open. Some office appointments had been made for me for my return, but in the meantime two other ophthalmologists had set up in Willowdale beside Dr. Somerville. Thus, there was practice-building to be done.

This part of the city had grown phenomenally since I had first visited and worked in a small private hospital called Bethesda twenty years before. This had been a large residence on spacious grounds which had been converted to a twenty-bed hospital associated with the training arm of the Missionary Health Institute. Then the village had been called Lansing. With the fusing of municipalities to form Metropolitan Toronto, Lansing had disappeared into North York, which was later to become a city in its own right. Bethesda Hospital had also been merged with the new North York General Hospital, and the grounds were now occupied by apartment buildings.

Newfoundland had changed me. There I had been needed, and I had worked very hard to meet those needs in Central Newfoundland and the Grenfell area. Now I was a tiny speck in a giant pool of people. Although I had relatives who were close, I was very conscious of my solitude, and I had not the long hours of work which had helped me to suppress my loneliness. Then I met Annelise May, who, as a Ph.D. in microbiology and biochemistry, was in charge of a private laboratory. Although I was fifty-nine, I was able to persuade her to marry me in 1974. We had our honeymoon in Paris, where I had never been. Somehow I could not get work out of my blood, even on my honeymoon, for we attended a Prevention of Blindness Conference there before going to Britain to meet her relatives in London, and then to Scotland, where my school and university days were spent. After returning to Toronto, Annelise continued with her professional work, as an inspector of laboratories for the govenment of Ontario, which she had taken after leaving the private laboratory. We were to continue in our own professions until the next project.

5 / *The North Calls Again*

To follow that star, no matter how hopeless, no matter how far....

Man from La Mancha

I WAS TO SPEND most of the seventies in Toronto with my practice there; however, in March 1978, advertisements appeared in medical magazines and daily papers endeavouring to recruit ophthalmologists for the Northwest Territories. Dr. Hugh Rose had been holding down this strenuous post for eight years and wanted to be relieved. Stanton Hospital now planned a department with two medical eye doctors as well as certified ophthalmic technicians. There were also to be increased hospital facilities with the beds and specialists' offices in one health centre.

While this was a similar challenge to that which had taken me to Newfoundland, it was different in one particular. In Newfoundland I had been alone and lonely, so work was a relief. Now I was re-married, and my wife, Annelise, had her Ph.D. in biochemistry, with years of experience in research, as well as clinical laboratory management and inspection. Perhaps the territorial health service could use the expertise we each offered. And so it was that at the end of April 1978 we flew up from Edmonton by Pacific Western jet to look things over at Yellowknife. It was already becoming quite warm, and the snow was melting from the rocky terrain. We were met at the airport by the Stanton Hospital administrator, Mr. Nelson McClelland, and later by Dr. Hugh Rose who introduced us to his office, his staff and some of the workings of his far-flung practice.

The Northwest Territories is an immense area of 1.3 million square miles which for years has been under jurisdiction of the

federal government in Ottawa, as it was when I visited Frobisher Bay in 1965. This great expanse, though rich in minerals and
other resources, still has only 46,000 people and has not reached
provincial status. A start had now been made to responsible
self-government by elected representatives meeting as a territorial council in Yellowknife. A federal civil servant, the commissioner, acted as vice-regent. The health services of the
territorial council ran the Stanton Yellowknife Hospital, the
H. H. Williams Hospital at Hay River, and the new health centre at Fort Smith. The hospital at Yellowknife was named after
Dr. Stanton, who for twenty-five years cared for the people in
the area as it changed from a mining town to the main city and
referral centre of the Mackenzie zone. It is the only hospital
with salaried specialists in various fields, although it must be
confessed that rarely, if ever, is a full medical establishment in
place. The primary care in Yellowknife and in Hay River is
given by family practitioners on a fee-for-service scale. Many of
them also provide service on a contract basis to the surrounding
areas still under the federal Department of Health and Welfare.

As we looked at the map on the office wall we traced the
limits of the territory which had to be serviced: south to the
Alberta border, east to Fort Smith, west to Nahanni, Fort Liard
and Wrigley, north to Holman Island and east through the Inuit
bases of Coppermine, Cambridge Bay, Gjoa Haven, Spence Bay
and Pelly Bay. These areas north of the treeline had to be serviced twice a year at the beginning and the end of winter,
before most of the people scattered to the forward camps—
called "going on the land."

South of the northern limit of tree growth lay the land of the
Indian, into which the white world had insinuated itself. The
first to enter were the great explorers who followed the rivers
and lakes, then prospectors and fur traders and missionaries:
they were all lonely people supplied by Hudson's Bay posts.
Then the finds of pitchblende and silver at Great Bear Lake, oil
at Norman Wells, gold in Yellowknife and lead and zinc in Pine
Point allowed the barge-and-tug port of Hay River to grow to
supply the others. Each find brought more miners, workers and
supply personnel. Contact with the Indian increased. Traders

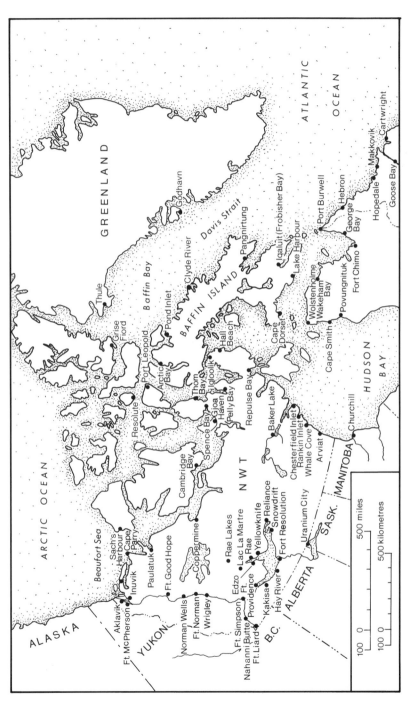

The Northwest Territories.

came bringing whisky and flour, which the meat-eating native could not metabolize well. Tuberculosis found a foothold and soon started to spread like a forest fire. Intermarriage introduced a fourth group into the already-tangled society—the Metis. Add to this the Indian who kept his former ways so that the Mackenzie Valley alone was home to six tribes—each with a different language not reduced to writing. Of these three, the Dogrib, Slavey and Chipewyan surround Great Slave Lake and find their way to the Yellowknife Hospital and clinics. Although the older generation is still divided by language and custom, the younger Indians, led by a new generation of chiefs, are finding common ground in their dealings with the federal government. The teaching of English in the schools has given them an advantage their fathers did not have.

While there is a great variety in the native people, the newcomers, especially in the larger mining centres such as Yellowknife, come from all over the world. The Chinese have an active community, especially in the food market and restaurant industries. Some German immigrants came to work in the mines and, after bringing over their families, became entrepreneurs in small businesses. As we looked around the office walls we found charts and folders of people in every walk of life, and almost all nations. All those who have passed through the eye service, whether in the settlements or in Yellowknife, have a file on the shelves. During all visits to the outstations, duplicate charts were made, one of which was kept in the nursing station, the other in the department's master file. Thus when a call came from Fort Liard about a patient with a painful red eye, it took only a minute to pull the chart. The symptoms were described by the nurse, and it was decided that the condition was probably a recurrence of iritis, for which he had been treated successfully two years before. As there would be no plane from Fort Liard for two days, the nurse was instructed to recommence the previous medication. Three options were available: The patient could continue with the treatment until the doctor from Fort Simpson visited in two weeks, or the patient could be transferred to Fort Simpson Hospital, or he could be sent to the base hospital in Yellowknife. The eye team was not due to visit Fort Liard for another two months.

Since it was virtually impossible for one person to cover the area adequately, we used paramedic personnel in the form of certified ophthalmic technicians (C.O.T.), who underwent extensive training and examination covering an approved course. Desmond Grant, C.O.T., was the first to assist Dr. Rose in his wide practice,[1] and as the result of this experience it was decided to try to develop a training course and to teach long-term residents in the North to care for those in isolated communities. Thus when Des Grant moved with his family to Edmonton, Kathe Burkhard, C.O.T., was hired to assist in the clinical work, and also to develop a two-year training program. Kathe was to prepare a training course for the new school envisaged to help N.W.T. residents become ophthalmic technicians. At the same time Bev Tarver, C.O.T., was hired to assist Dr. Rose, particularly in the travel clinics.

Before being shown round the Stanton Hospital, we had an excellent buffet lunch at the eight-storey Explorer Hotel, where we stayed during our visit. There was a generous sprinkling of service uniforms (some Russian) reflecting the fact that the search was still continuing for parts of a satellite which had plunged to Earth and probably lay buried in Great Slave Lake.

As we drove to the hospital we passed high-rise offices and apartment buildings, many housing government personnel, which formed the core of the new Yellowknife. By contrast, the hospital seemed to be low-profile and tired. While functioning adequately, some departments were obviously overcrowded. The furnace system, which had to battle so hard during the long winter months, had to be coaxed along. The hospital also had a serious structural defect. It had been built in a hurry when the previous one was destroyed by fire, and part of its foundation had mistakenly been built on permafrost, which subsided to such a degree that a ramp was required to connect it to the section based on rock. The municipal and territorial governments were keen to see the new hospital built, but the federal government, which used many beds for the care of its

Indian and Inuit wards, was hesitant about assuming its share of the cost.

After leaving the hospital we were driven to the old Yellowknife, which had grown up in response to gold strikes in the late 1930s, and another in 1945. We visited Weaver and Devore, the general suppliers who had equipped many a gold-digging operation and a host of prospectors. We passed the float plane base which forms the home of the charter service to all parts of the North. On a crag at the peak of the rocky peninsula around which the planes huddle is the Bush Pilot's Monument. This is to honour the men who in the early days flew over and charted the wilderness. Then we crossed the small bridge to Latham Island and Rainbow Valley—the latter home to most of the Indian inhabitants whose multicolored dwellings dot the peninsula jutting into Great Slave Lake. The rainbow painted on the end of the school enhances the picture. The other Dogrib Indian village, Detah, can be reached across the harbour by ice road in winter, but requires a long trip around the bay in the summer months.

The next day in a conference with me, the administrator emphasized a defect in the eye service identified in a survey by the Central and Eastern Arctic Health Services (CEAHS). In April 1977, CEAHS had reported:

> In nearly every community visited during the data-gathering portion of this study, comments were made by community council members, residents and nurses about difficulties in this field. Services were sporadic, and some communities had not been visited in this specialty area during the past two years. When the specialists did come, sometimes there was insufficient notice given to those people out hunting and/or trapping so they could arrange to travel into town to see the specialist. There were many complaints about the length of time required to receive glasses and the adjustments required to obtain a reasonable fitting. Complaints about the quality of frames were common. Repairs for broken glasses and frames are stated to be very difficult to arrange and there are also lengthy service delays.
>
> A way must be found to correct the deficiencies in this service area. However, such factors as weather conditions, transpor-

tation, and the availability of specialty services must be recognized.[2]

The Legislative Assembly had taken note of this report, and was willing to expand the eye service by two ophthalmologists and start a school for ophthalmic technicians. Students were to be recruited from the N.W.T., and a minimum of ten years' residence was obligatory. This was passed by the commissioner and executive on January 12, 1978. The advertisement which I had seen in Toronto was the result of this decision.

The administrator offered my wife and me posts as laboratory coordinator and zone ophthalmologist, respectively. We decided to have someone look after my practice in Toronto from August to December. Annelise was particularly excited. She had come North primarily to please me, but had fallen under its spell and the challenge it offered.

When we returned to Toronto we began preparing for the four-month trip. The biggest task was to find a doctor who could care for my practice during my absence. This was accomplished just before we were due to leave. We had arranged to rent an apartment from the Yellowknife hospital, but it had only the hard furniture and appliances. We had to take sheets, towels, dishes, pots and pans and clothing for both summer and winter. While the temperature can become very hot during the long summer days when tropical clothing is appropriate, it can also drop to minus forty in the winter.

We read up about the journey, and were happy to have driving hints for car protection: the Mackenzie Highway in the territories was gravel, so windshields and headlights could fall victims to flying stones. We were able to find plastic covers for the headlights, but in Ontario no one seemed to know how to make a protective shield for a gas tank. We decided to have some of these things done on the way. In the middle of August 1978 we drove the station wagon, loaded as full as the law would allow, with two very heavy suitcases jammed with reference books on the roof rack, to start our western journey. We designated it a holiday, so there was no desire to break records. As neither of us had travelled in northern Ontario, it was an

exploratory trip. We enjoyed the scenery north of Lake Super-
ior, and marvelled at the size of the province. We had only
driven partially across Ontario, but still it took 1,200 miles to
reach its western boundary near Kenora.

Having seen the prairie only from the plane and train, it
was a new feeling to drive the flat expanse covering most of
Manitoba and Saskatchewan. Before reaching Winnipeg we took
an instructive detour to Steinbach, where the Mennonite
museum provided background about this group inhabiting
much of the area, and exhibited pictures of the early days of
pioneering in the West. Now everything seemed so prosperous
in the area. Could it be that the museum was not only a tourist
attraction, but served also to remind people of their roots? The
museum stood guard against the erosion of the religious and
pioneer fibre which so often follows success.

Winnipeg, what memories it stirred! In 1948, just thirty years
before, this was the city where I had taken the examination giving me the title of Licentiate of the Medical Council of Canada.

Our next stop was Saskatoon, where it was my wife's turn
to reminisce. The last time she had been in that city was 1967,
when she had given a lecture in the Department of Microbiology of the University of Saskatchewan. We had a look at the
university and visited a reconstructed street of a Prairie
town—part of Saskatchewan's attempt to remind itself of its
heritage and roots.

We pushed along the Yellowhead Highway, which takes its
name from one of the most famous guides of the early days.
This remarkable blond man (hence the name Yellowhead or
Tête Jaune) had led many caravans along the same trail into
and over the Rockies. He had left his name there too, as the
Tête Jaune Cache. Finally we reached Edmonton, the last major
city on our trip. We continued west along the Yellowhead, and
then swung north on the Mackenzie Highway. We soon found
ourselves on the direct path to much of Alberta's wealth. It was
hard, driving on this two-lane road pursued by giant diesel
trucks loaded with construction and pipeline equipment—all
trying for the fastest turnaround time. We were glad to stop at
Fox Creek, where we obtained the only available bed in the

motels which form much of its main street. During the week, all the rooms were taken by construction workers.

Fox Creek, though only a village, announces its greatness with a huge sign stating it is the centre of the largest natural gas field in the world. During the night giant diesels ran continuously in front of the restaurant, for already the days were shortening and there was much to do before winter came.

At Valleyview the Mackenzie Highway continues north while the highway to Grande Prairie, Dawson Creek and Alaska turns off. Suddenly we felt alone, as the heavy traffic took the other road and we could make our own speed toward Peace River. We still had a long way to go, as Yellowknife is almost 1,000 miles north of Edmonton. The road was well-paved throughout most of Alberta, but near Steen River there had been problems. Ruts were deep, and we were glad we had put extra-heavy loadleveler shocks on the vehicle. We were in no danger of being stuck, as road construction equipment was standing by. Dr. Rose had lost his muffler in that area on his way south, but fortunately ours was still undamaged. The road soon resumed its good quality, and we passed Indian Cabins where the last gas pumps south of the sixtieth parallel were to be found.

A large sign announced our arrival at the Northwest Territories. A giant three-legged polar bear, the symbol of the region, reminded us that there were no more boundaries to cross before we reached the North Pole. Hot coffee was served at the Welcome Station, and the people were friendly. This is often the case: the more rugged the land and climate, the warmer the inhabitants. Cities are often the coldest places on God's Earth.

Road conditions became worse; gravelled and dusty. Headlights were on as a safety precaution, as one car travelling behind another vehicle would not be seen in the cloud of dust. We learned to slow down when other cars—and especially trucks—came. Certain sections were designated dust-free, where the road had been oiled and posted as passing zones.

Apart from these limitations, the area was attractive. There were three beautiful waterfalls on the Hay River just beside the

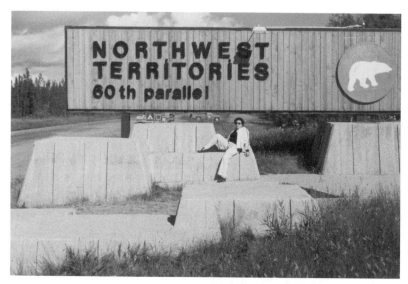

Sign at 60th parallel with three-legged bear.

road, with picnic areas well cared for. Car licence plates from Alberta, British Columbia and even the northern United States showed that this was a fisherman's paradise. At Enterprise, a gas station and restaurant marked the junction of the road running along the south side of Great Slave Lake to Hay River and Fort Smith. We turned the other way toward Fort Simpson and then north once more, toward Fort Providence and Yellowknife. We reached the bank of the mighty Mackenzie River. Although it still had more than 1,000 miles to flow before reaching the Beaufort Sea, it was over a mile wide. We crossed by ferry, which had to struggle against the cross-current flowing at more than ten knots. By the time we had eaten at Fort Providence, it was well into the afternoon. There was still plenty of daylight; in that northern summer we could have gone further, but we knew this last lap to Yellowknife was 200 miles without service stations on a gravel road. So we stayed the night in the modern, well-appointed Snowshoe Inn.

The next day was Sunday so we did not stir too early, and were able to have a look round the pretty hamlet set up on the cliff overlooking the Mackenzie. We passed the ubiquitous

Hudson's Bay store, the school and the nursing station. At the end of the road was a white wooden Roman Catholic church. We joined the worshippers, mainly Slavey Indian people, for the Grey Nuns had founded and still carried on a school and mission, one of the oldest in the territories. There was a sense of bereavement in the service led by a French-Canadian priest, for the Pope had just died, and his successor had not yet been named. Although not sharing with the congregation in religious affiliation, we could heartily share in the prayers that guidance should be given in the choice of a new leader. Certainly the world needed a man of strength, integrity and wisdom in a society bent on re-evaluating all its political and moral tenets.

After a quick snack we turned the wagon once more toward our goal, and arrived without incident and without having to use the spare gasoline. We found the keys for our apartment at the hospital switchboard, with a note of welcome from the administrator. We were soon unpacking to start a new temporary nest in the North.

The windows faced west. In the evening the sun was very bright, but ended with a glorious sunset. Every evening was shorter by six minutes, until we came home in the dark. It was becoming distinctly colder too, and then the first snow fell. This quickly melted, but the next stayed. Winter was beginning.

As we kept busy and well-wrapped, the cooler temperatures were invigorating. Every morning before the national news on the radio there was a "Mackenzie Round-up," which kept us informed of doings in our zone. Ice was forming on the river, but the ferry at Fort Providence was open. Trucks were running frequently from Edmonton bringing extra supplies, for the stores in Yellowknife were stocking up for winter. People were betting on whether the crossing would close earlier or later than normal, and how long it would be until the ice bridge formed. It seemed such a short time ago since we had been able to play tennis in the evening without lights—now we saw the sun only at lunch and on weekends. The setting orb was still glorious, however. This cycle continued until the day we saw two sunsets.

A clinic for Cambridge Bay had been scheduled for the first week in December. As we were soon to return to Ontario, and my wife had finished her assignment, she offered to help. Our jet was due to leave about noon. We had not realized that the plane first went to Resolute, high up in the Arctic. It was a smooth flight, and as we watched the sky turned crimson and the sun seemed to die a glorious death. We plunged forward into the Arctic night, broken only by our flashing navigation lights and a giant moon so low it seemed at our wingtip.

At Resolute the co-pilot visited the passengers, and as we were reading he stopped near us. "I know you," he said. I could not place him, although the face was vaguely familiar. I said I was going to Cambridge Bay to hold an eye clinic for the Stanton Yellowknife Hospital. "That's it," he said. "I saw you in the hospital." Then I remembered. He had taken some hunters into Great Bear Lake in his own plane, and while stowing antlers in the luggage compartment had caught a tip in his eye and lacerated an upper lid. Now with his lid well-healed, and in his uniform, he looked a different man. He wanted Annelise and me to come up front. We made our way through the cargo section to the cockpit, where two seats were available behind the crew. Soon we were climbing to six miles high. It was very dark—it had been pitch black in Resolute since 1 p.m.—but suddenly the sky was a blaze of red once more. We had been travelling rapidly south and had again caught the sun blushingly retiring for the night. In a moment it was over, and we started our descent toward a spot of light which grew into the runway and community of Cambridge Bay.

On December 21 we left Yellowknife for Toronto. We had thought we would sell the station wagon and fly back, but we did not realize that vehicles which have been exposed to the salt on winter roads in Ontario do not attract buyers in the West. Also, we had not calculated on the exodus to family reunions and warmer climes which takes place over the winter break. Flights were booked solid many months in advance. We started loading the car early, but it was slow and very cold work at thirty-five degrees below zero. The plastic dustcovers for dresses and suits shivered and cracked. The apartment seemed to take forever to clear and clean. A Transair plane, in which some of our friends were leaving for Christmas, took off overhead and seemed to mock us as it headed for Winnipeg and Toronto. How we wished we could have joined the flight!

A friend had given us a good breakfast, so we suffered no hunger pangs leaving just after noon. With two or three hours of daylight left, we drove steadily the first sixty miles past the community and nursing station at Rae-Edzo, and started the 130-mile stretch to Fort Providence. Although we knew the ice bridge was open, there was essentially no traffic. Even with the heater on full, the windows were fogged up, but the windshield was clear and the wirestrips on the rear window kept it mostly frost-free. Through the snow cloud behind us I could see headlights rapidly approaching. The other driver obviously knew the road—probably a trapper making tracks for home. Without slackening speed I pulled slightly to the side. With a flash of red tail light the other car was swallowed in a cloud of snow, so the driver probably did not realize that the heavy snow had caught my right front wheel, wrenching my steering. We were stuck in deep snow in the ditch about seventy miles from Fort Providence. Too late, the admonition, given by a friend before we left Yellowknife to stop to let others pass, was recalled.

There was nothing we could do. We were at a steep angle. Digging would not free us even if we had four-wheel drive. It seemed appropriate to pray, which we did. We hoped the snowplow we had passed earlier might come over the brow of the hill. Little did we know that we had also passed the work camp where this vehicle turned off.

Travellers on the lonely road are supposed to report their destinations to the Royal Canadian Mounted Police prior to leaving, and check in again at the point of arrival. Although we had reported our departure from Yellowknife, we discovered later that the officer at Fort Providence did not know of our call, so it would have been a long time before a search party came. I had arranged to hold a clinic at Hay River the next day, so if we did not show, the hospital would probably contact the police. Meanwhile there was nothing to do except wait. We wrapped ourselves in sleeping bags, as the car was getting cold, and we had candles, which when lit can keep a car warm enough for survival.

While we pondered the truth of the old maxim, "More haste, less speed," we noticed lights in the distance. A giant diesel belonging to Byers Transport drew up alongside. It looked like a train, with its long trailer and pup. "Don't worry," said the driver, "I do this three times a week. I've even pulled out a snowplow with this rig." Sure enough, he took out a heavy chain, fastened it to our car and pulled us out. Then he helped us clear the engine of snow. The engine, still not completely cold, started easily. As daylight was failing we were glad our headlights had suffered no damage, and with their help travelled the last seventy miles to our goal.

We have not found out why it was given the name Fort Providence, but possibly the earliest visitor may have had a deliverance such as ours. It was only when we were having dinner in the motel restaurant, and met some of the Byers' workers, that we heard of the miracle of timing we had experienced. The ice bridge was still not firm enough to carry trucks, so only one big load of urgent supplies was being sent to the south bank of the Mackenzie River each day. The contents were transferred to another truck on the north shore by helicopter. The vehicle which had rescued us left in the afternoon to supply Yellowknife, returning during the night to be ready for another trip the next day. As we left the next morning for Hay River, we saw the helicopter being readied to start its day's work.

Traversing the ice bridge was not hard, provided the rules were obeyed. The "bridge" was a well-marked strip of carefully groomed and periodically checked ice about a mile east of the regular ferry crossing. As the weight of each vehicle created a wave ahead of it, it was mandatory to travel in low gear at five miles an hour. If the speed was too great, the wave would strike the shore too quickly and the rebound could crack the ice. We were soon on the "dicey" road to Hay River, where I had an afternoon consultation clinic.

The next morning a telephone call woke us. My secretary in Toronto was calling to say a teaching post was available for

Annelise at Ryerson Institute if we could reach Toronto by January 3.

Driving was hazardous, but we reached Edmonton in safety and left on Christmas Day, travelling via Calgary and the Trans-Canada Highway to Ontario.

6 / An Open Door at Sixty-four

Bring the good old bugle boys. We'll sing another song.

Marching through Georgia, 1864

I T W A S G O O D to be home, but neither my wife nor I could forget our time in the North. When Annelise's session was over, the door was open for our return: there was much work for both of us to do.

Besides the clinical work, there was the challenge of training northerners to work as technicians in the territories. But what about age? As we were considering what to do, my sixty-fourth birthday came. There was no point in leaving a practice for government service if in a few months I would be classed as redundant, as industry, and even various levels of government, were wont to do to employees. We were assured that forced retirement could be postponed if we were fit enough. Both of us had been given good health—we could play tennis, hike, climb mountain trails, and even cross-country ski, provided these things were done in moderation. With no disability, why should we hold back?

Last of all, there had been no great response to the many advertisements placed in medical magazines for someone to hold the position on a long-term basis. This was necessary if there was to be a training scheme for paramedics as planned. Fortunately the clinical care of eye cases in the Mackenzie Zone was being carried by Dr. R. Kukreja, F.R.C.S.(C), but he did not want to commit himself to the two-year minimum period required to pass the first class through the curriculum. As there was provision for two ophthalmologists, we decided to return, provided my wife could be adequately stimulated by work in the laboratory field. This was arranged, and we started to make plans for disposal of the practice, apartment and office.

I had always felt that God had a plan for every life, and it began to look as if this challenge of the North was part of this. An incident came at this time which reinforced this belief. We went one Sunday evening to a church in a part of Toronto with which we were not familiar, where a friend was to sing. The church was honouring some of its senior members, and the minister chose to read a portion of Joshua 14. It was the story of Caleb, who, as a forty-year-old warrior, was sent to spy out the land. Now, forty years later, still fit at eighty years, he says, "Give me this mountain, which I was promised."[1] There was rugged terrain and giants. But his courage was as great as the challenge, and he got his wish. The minister then spoke of some people who had done their greatest work *after* they had become senior citizens: Churchill and Colonel Saunders were two examples. We came away with the thought that, with spirit, health and God's help, age was no deterrent.

Things started to roll. We were able to sell our building. An ophthalmologist took over the practice and the charts, and suddenly we were free. August 10, 1979 saw the moving van pull out of our driveway. Shortly afterward, we journeyed north to Owen Sound, then across Manitoulin Island to join the Trans-Canada Highway on its way west. From Edmonton we decided to avoid the heavy trucks on the Mackenzie Highway so we travelled north to the village of Slave Lake, where we rested at a motel run by the Sawbridge Indian band. It was comfortable and efficiently operated with a good restaurant. It was reassuring to see a group of natives operating effectively in what is usually a white man's world. Turning west we were able to reach the Mackenzie Highway south of Peace River.

Leaving the plateau, we descended to the great valley through which runs the Peace River. This rises from the mountains near Dawson Creek, receives the waters of the Smoky River at the town of Peace River, and continues north to skirt Lake Athabasca and change its name to the Slave River. Finally it enters Great Slave Lake near Fort Resolution, and leaves that body of water as the Mackenzie River which we were to cross for the third time the next day. After that there was only the dusty road to Yellowknife and the start of a new challenge. We had burned our bridges, we could only go forward.

Annelise and I ended up staying for nearly seven years in Yellowknife, so it was a good thing we enjoyed both the life and the people. Though there was plenty to keep us occupied in the clinical field in the hospital, and also the travel clinics, the actual start of the school took much planning, as it was in many ways different from any previously attempted.

I had not been in Yellowknife long when the phone rang. The caller was on long distance but did not hold long enough to have the secretary reach me. She left a message: "Have Dr. Gillan call Dr. Cass in Fort Smith."

When I dutifully returned the call, the voice on the line gave every indication of aggression. "So they are bringing doctors over from Britain to look after my area of the North, are they?"

Evidently Elizabeth Cass had discovered my British degrees and had concluded that I had arrived directly from the U.K. Actually I had come to Canada eight years before her, but she still considered the Mackenzie Zone her area. It was true that she had worked in it for years, until her employer, the federal government, had retired her because of their policy on age. She had never forgiven Dr. Rose, my predecessor, for having usurped her rightful domain. This situation was going to require "the soft answer to turn away wrath" (Proverbs 15. 1).

"Don't you know me? I've been working in the east for years, and spent time in Newfoundland and Labrador," I said smoothly.

"I don't know much about those areas," she replied, her voice losing its edge.

"I heard you lecture at the Pan-American Congress in Montreal. I even wrote to have a copy of your talk."

Knowing that she often came to Yellowknife to see friends, I suggested that she call and meet me on her next visit. As she knew everyone of importance, and had spent her life pulling strings, I knew the call might come at any time when there was an empty seat on a returning government plane.

In about a week, the call came. Elizabeth was spending the weekend with her special friends Dr. and Mrs. Pearse O'Donoghue, long-time residents of Yellowknife. I suggested that we go for a meal together. Being a gourmet cook, she knew exactly where to go. She chose the "Gold Range," where she knew the chef, who could produce the best Chinese food.

I was surprised at how frail she was. She claimed that her weakness was due to a furnace which was faulty and leaked carbon monoxide. She was only the shell of the woman who had been able to face off the bureaucracy of the British army brass and the Canadian federal government. Over dinner and on several occasions after that I came to piece together her remarkable career.

Emily Elizabeth Cass was born in 1904 in England, and educated in Cheltenham Ladies College. She obtained her MRCS and LRCP in 1927 followed by her MBBS in 1928 at St. Mary's Hospital Medical School. By 1935, having worked in four hospitals, she was chief clinical assistant, Moorfields Eye Hospital and St. Mary's Hospital, Paddington. Between 1934 and 1939, she published eleven articles on various ophthalmological subjects and had been awarded the Research Scholarship of London University for research in strabismus (turn in the eyes). The same year—as she was fluent in Spanish—she was invited by the governments of Argentina and Brazil to give a course of seven lectures on the etiology and treatment of strabismus.

In 1940, she was appointed a senior ophthalmologist in the Royal Army Medical Corps with the rank of major—the only woman so honoured. In 1943 she was transferred to Gibraltar after attending a course in plastic surgery in East Grinstead for three months. She continued there until 1955 as ophthalmic surgeon to the military and colonial hospitals, taking time to lecture in Spanish in Madrid, Seville and Cuba.

In 1956, she emigrated to Canada, was appointed an ophthalmologist to the Department of Health and Welfare, and was transferred to the Northwest Territories two years later. There she worked intensely to bring care to a part of Canada often forgotten by the medical establishment.

She was never recognized by the Royal College of Surgeons, which has acknowledged people with less accomplishments by time-honoured "grandfathering." Was it because she was a woman, or that her tongue was sharper than the Graefe knife she used? Was it perhaps because the college did not want to be reminded that this woman had brought an altruism and dedication to a part of Canada that was at that time medically Third World?

Dr. Cass was tall and strongly boned, and she demonstrated her physical prowess with a London University purple for rowing in 1927 and Villars Cup for bobsleighing in 1932. She had need of her physical capacity, as she often had to take her bulky equipment by bush plane or dog team to remote settlements. In only about four of the settlements were there hotels, so most trips found her housed in schools or homes.

She recorded having to spend the night in teepees when "weathered in." She had a working knowledge of several Indian and Inuit dialects and recorded legends, songs and folklore of the North, for which she received the Commissioner's Award in 1968.[2]

In spite of the difficulties in travel, Dr. Cass kept notes and statistics on which she could base the twenty papers she presented to the eight medical societies to which she belonged, and at the circumpolar conferences she attended regularly. Dr. Cass also kept in active touch with many senior ophthalmologists all over the world, and in Yellowknife in 1970 representatives of thirteen countries gathered to form the International Society of Geographic Ophthalmology, of which she was elected president.

This society has now grown to have local secretariats in twenty-two countries from as far away as New Zealand, the U.S.S.R. and North and South America. Well-known ophthalmologists such as Arnold Sorsby of the U.K., G. Palameris of Greece, Henrik Forsius of Finland and many other professors familiar to ophthalmologists take active roles. In 1970, Dr. Cass was also honoured with the Order of Canada for her pioneer service in the North.

But she was also very much a woman. At receptions she would often wear Dior creations. She was never happier than in the kitchen cooking gourmet meals. Her book, *Spanish Cooking*, was published in 1957 and had its third printing in 1970.[3]

Finally, retired against her will by the federal health service because of her age, she set up private practice in Fort Smith, N.W.T. There, in spite of her long record of honours, she endured the final humiliation of not being able to bill the territorial health insurance as a specialist because she had not sat the exams of the Royal College of Surgeons.

She died in 1980 in Fort Smith, among the Indian and Metis community who loved and honoured her. She was remembered too by the International Society of Geographic Ophthalmologists over which she had presided. At each conference there is an Elizabeth Cass Memorial Lecture. As she had died impecunious, the society, working with the local legion, purchased a stone.

At the ceremony a tribute from the International Society was read which ended: "Emily Elizabeth Cass, as members of that world which you tried to unite in fraternal bonds, we pay tribute to your memory as we place this stone."

When we began our time in Yellowknife the presence of Dr. Kukreja was of great assistance, as we could divide the work in the Stanton Hospital as well as in the H. H. Williams Hospital in Hay River, where the physicians in charge arranged for cases to be seen by us monthly. There were also hospitals with physicians in charge in the smaller communities of Fort Simpson and Cambridge Bay. Each of these had satellite communities, some with nurses in charge, and other hamlets which the nurse and physician visited at set intervals.

A great deal of effort was necessary to organise this travel program. Some of the larger centres were served by Pacific Western Airlines using jet aircraft, and Northwest Territorial Airways which had scheduled flights using four-engine Lockheed Electras to Frobisher Bay and Winnipeg, as well as the slower DC-3 serving northern centres. Some areas were served by smaller companies using scheduled flights with de Havilland Otters or Beavers with their excellent short take-off and landing capabilities. Some of the hamlets could only be reached by chartering small aircraft. All this flying was necessary because

Yellowknife is at the end of the Mackenzie Highway. In the winter some of the mines can bring heavy equipment over the frozen muskeg and lakes, but these winter roads had no benefit to the eye service as the trucks were only for company use and ran when load and travel conditions were suitable. Most often they did not supply settlements.

No matter how carefully scheduling was arranged, the final determining factor was the weather. Even when a flight had started, the weather could change unpredictably en route. On one such occasion, Jeffrey Oxler, a certified ophthalmic technician, was returning from Fort Simpson when fog set in. It was a chartered flight from Providence Air, owned and operated by a long-time resident of Fort Providence who had taken part in many searches for downed planes. Fortunately he was able to pick up the reflection of the Mackenzie River when he flew low enough. By following its course east to his home base, he was able to find the highway at the ferry crossing and follow it to Yellowknife, where the runways were clear enough for landing. Most often the flights were not in areas where such definite signposts existed, then it was by the well-worn seat of the pilot's pants, and most of all by God's grace, which fortunately was extended to all our staff during our stay in the North.

Because of the possibility of a plane crashing or having to make a forced landing, all of us who had to go on travel clinics were required to take a survival course. This consisted of lectures and films showing how to signal from the ground using the international code of three equally placed distinct fires—the main one for warmth, and two subsidiaries which could be lit from the first if the drone of a plane were heard. We were also taught how to use the wire from the fuselage to make snares for small animals, and how to make nets to pass under ice holes to catch fish. We were to take Arctic sleeping bags or space blankets of folding foil as well as a small box or tin containing fish hooks, nails, needle and thread, compass, insect repellant (very important for summer use), a small mirror to signal aircraft, stay-dry matches or cigarette lighter and strong cord. Each of the bush planes was supposed to carry first-aid equipment and a weapon for defence against attacking animals.

Another interesting character I met, who left his mark on the North (and who has recently died) was Ernie Lyall—E5.1. Ernie was born Caucasian, but the figure "E" labelled him an Eskimo or Inuit.

I first met Ernie in Spence Bay, N.W.T. on March 18, 1980, for this is the record he made autographing my copy of the book he had just written. When I saw that he was on my list for eye examination, I purchased his story *An Arctic Man, Sixty-five Years in Canada's North*.[4] When I asked for his signature this is what he wrote: "To Graham Gillan, the man who looked me in the eye, so hopefully I will now be able to read this book."

His weather-beaten face testified to the long time he had spent in the North, under winter weather conditions of intense cold and long hours of sunlight in the summer.

By judicious protection from glare his corneas had not shown signs of disease, but he was now suffering from early senile cataracts, and the book he had written was transcribed from tapes given to Hurtig Publishers in Edmonton.

With his usual frankness he states: "The main reason I decided to do a book about my life in the north is that I finally got fed up with all the baloney in so many books written about the north." (13)

He was particularly critical of Farley Mowat's book *The Snow Walker*,[5] which mentions Ernie's name but, said Ernie, did not get the facts straight. Ernie would know—he was an R.C.M.P. interpreter throughout the trial of Soosie's killers.[6] He also pointed out that he had heard people calling Mr. Farley Mowat "Mr. Hardly Know-It."(227) Naturally, residents in the North are sensitive about having their lifestyle misrepresented, or their feelings trampled, by people who make a living from writing books about them.

Ernie was born in Labrador in 1910, between Makkovik and Hopedale, but his father of Scottish descent left the Hudson's Bay Company and went to work at the store of the Moravian Mission at Port Burwell, a small island just off the coast of the northern tip of Labrador.

Most of the Lyall family of nineteen children were scattered along Labrador, and I was able to tell Ernie that I had cared for some of his relatives when I used to work there in the 1960s. Ernie had long since lost track of most of them because his pathway was west, while they remained in Labrador.

Ernie Lyall joined the Hudson's Bay Company after school in St. John's, Newfoundland. He and several other clerks signed on for $20 a month and board. On their first trip North, the ship ran aground, but as there were plenty of lifeboats as well as some fishing craft transported as deck cargo, all escaped. Because of the delay and bad weather he was not able to reach his first assignment at Cape Smith, but had to spend most of the winter of 1917–18 at Wolstenholme.

The North is rough survival country and there were plenty of these stories in Ernie's book, but surprisingly it is really a love story.

It was in Arctic Bay that Ernie found Nipisha, the eldest daughter of Kavavouk, one of the characters in Farley Mowat's book. Ernie's Inuit had become quite fluent by that time; Kavavouk had been a leader of the Inuit at Cape Dorset, and had been a port servant for the company for many years, and as such he moved to Arctic Bay.

Nipisha was a house maid in the staff house there, and Ernie and she met often. While the company building was being finished, Ernie fell off a ladder and hit his elbow against a rock. The bruising was so severe that he was not able to use it, and Nipisha would bring his meals. Later they used to go rabbit and ptarmigan hunting together, or just walking. He was also impressed by the fact that she could handle a dogsled when the snows came.

Ernie becomes rather embarrassed at this stage and says he is not writing a romance, but he sums up: "Nipisha was a fine girl, and after nearly forty-two years together I think she's a fine woman, so I guess you'll just have to be satisfied with that." (102)

It is probable that she was never able to read this tribute, for when I examined Nipisha's eyes I discovered that she did not seem to be able to read English, but Ernie was nearby to translate. She knew of his devotion, however, as when the challenge came he was able to show it by his number, E5.1.

In 1940, Ernie was in Fort Ross when a new manager came and wanted to send Ernie to Arctic Bay without his wife. This he refused to do. Heslop, the manager, didn't think he was serious when Ernie said that he was not going to leave his pregnant wife—he would resign.

Resignation was no easy thing in the Arctic, for it was immediately pointed out to Ernie that no white man was allowed to make a living by hunting and trapping in the Fort Ross area. Presumably the Hudson's Bay Company authorities thought that he was the one trapped.

Not so! Ernie had the language, had developed the skills, and had his father-in-law, the most skilful Inuit in the area, to help him. The *Nascopie*, a Hudson's Bay Company supply ship, was at the harbour with Major McKeand, a local government official, aboard. When McKeand heard the problem, he told Ernie, "As long as you live as an Eskimo—do as Eskimos do, trap as Eskimos do, and consider yourself as an Eskimo— you can stay and trap and hunt in the Northwest Territories." (119) Ernie immediately became an official Eskimo on the register.

In 1941, the federal government decided to stop the confusion in Inuit names. These were often changed and anglicized by missionaries and the R.C.M.P., so the spelling could be variable even when no change was intended. Probably the idea came from the dog tags issued to military personnel. The Eskimo were therefore numbered according to the area of residence and given numbered discs to carry. The E5 informed the initiated that he was from the area of Fort Ross or Pond Inlet and the numer "1" showed that he was the first to be tagged by the R.C.M.P. in that area.

To many, this idea of numbering seemed to lower the Inuit in their own, and others', eyes. I remember feeling that way when I visited Frobisher Bay in 1965. There must have been enough pressure, for the government started Project Surname giving all the people in the communities a second name. This caused confusion again, and most people realize it was a mistake. I should have remembered that from 1940–45, when I had carried British army officer number 159685, which I had to remember in case I was captured during World War II. Now all

Canadians are numbers as far as government computers are concerned.

Ernie, throughout his lifetime, acted as a bridge between the culture of the North and South with the help of the R.C.M.P., government officials and touring judges, for whom he acted as interpreter. Perhaps a suitable epitaph might be: "He tried to bring understanding and cut bureaucratic red tape."

Ernie did get his cataract operated upon by my successor, Dr. Smith, and was able to read again with his intraocular lens. He had seen much change in the Arctic of his youth, from the first aid given by Hudson's Bay Company traders and a few Mounties who travelled by ships in the summer and dog team in emergency winter trips, to a network of nursing stations with telephone contacts to specialists. There are visits by medical practitioners, and specialists in the major disciplines. The sky is the highway, for routine as well as emergency care.

Ernie believed that there was no prospect for the young in the local communities of the North—wide diffusion was necessary. His family carried out his belief, for they are scattered from Newfoundland to Yellowknife while Nipisha, their mother, was on the Territorial Committee on Land Claims. Of the other family members, two are homemakers, two are special constables with the R.C.M.P., one with a native Eskimo-owned co-op which is rivalling the Hudson's Bay Company in service to the North. Another has worked in oil and gas in the North, and one son, Bill, was elected to the Northwest Territorial Council and helped to shape legislation consistent with northern aspirations. Rest in peace, E5.1, your work is carrying on.

While extra classes, as well as St. John's Ambulance training, was added to the course our students were to take, 1980 came but we still had no class to teach. Being a government school, there were many interested departments which formed our advisory committee for the Ophthalmic Medical Assistant Training Program under the chairmanship of Mr. Nelson McClelland, Stanton Hospital administrator, who was to provide the space and teaching personnel.

The Department of Education wanted to have a say in what was being taught. They had formed Thebacha College in Fort

Smith, and had in view an Arctic College for even higher education for students from the Northwest Territories, which I will discuss later in this chapter. The territorial government's Department of Personnel wanted to screen the students to make sure the condition originally laid down that applicants must have been in the territories ten years was fulfilled. Health services in the territories were being slowly turned over from the federal government (which was still responsible for native care) to the territorial Department of Health; each had to have a say.

As usual, a budget had to be struck, and each of the interested groups had to provide funding. Although the Department of Personnel had chosen the three students, the program could not start until this funding was in place. All that came together in March 1980, when I was told the school would have to be functioning by the end of April, the end of the fiscal year, or there would be a delay of another year for re-budgeting.

The announcement of a start-up date could not have come at a worse time as far as the eye clinic was concerned, for we were in the midst of changes ourselves. Dr. Kukreja had left for the U.S., while Kathe Burkhard, having finished the draft of courses for the school, had left to plan and teach eye care in Haiti. To take her place as a clinical supervisor we had contacted Colonel Robert Forgie of the National Defence Hospital in Ottawa. We knew he had been training senior paramedics in the services in a two-year course in ophthalmology. Colonel Forgie had been active in the Joint Commission of Allied Health Professionals in Ophthalmology (JCAHPO), which registered those who graduated as ophthalmic assistants, technicians and technologists. Our advisory committee felt that to gain credibility, our school would have to be recognised by this body. A diploma from them would entitle our graduates to work with ophthalmologists throughout Canada and the U.S.

Colonel Forgie knew the man we needed—Sgt. Richard (Dick) Bryan. He had completed his course after being a paramedic with years of experience—including time with peacekeeping forces in the Middle East. Having attained the rank of sergeant, and unable to obtain commissioned officer status in his field, he was willing to leave the service. Fortunately he had been interviewed to take Kathe's place, but had not been released from his duties at Cold Lake, Alberta. Before Dick Bryan could reach us, our first three students arrived. Between our clinical cases, which we scheduled widely, Jeff Oxler started the class on optics while I taught anatomy of the eye and orbit. My wife was able to teach biology for the first few weeks. With the arrival of Dick Bryan our clinical load was relieved, and, as we had fulfilled our terms, we could claim our budget as a functioning school, and advertise for a clinical instructor.

Again Col. Forgie was able to assist us, as another of the servicemen he had trained planned to enter civilian life. Sgt. John (Jack) Clarke joined us in mid-1980, and proved to be an excellent choice. With their non-commissioned officer experience, both our ex-servicemen were used to performing in an organized and disciplined manner, and expected the same from their juniors. Dick Bryan took over running the office and arranging visits to our far-flung communities. Jack Clarke accepted the responsibility of primary tutor of the students, and their guidance through practical skills. Because of this teamwork, my duties were mainly medical and surgical care of patients in Stanton Hospital, teaching medical ophthalmology and general supervision of the outstations and hospitals on a regular schedule.

In 1981, the school was inspected by the Canadian Medical Association. One of the inspectors was Dr. Gordon Harris, President of the Canadian Ophthalmological Society. In 1953, as a newly graduated (and newly married) physician, he had been employed by the federal government to care for the Dogrib Indians at Rae.

In those days, there was a seventy-two bed hospital there that was fully occupied by tuberculosis patients, except for a few that were reserved for obstetrics and emergency care. Nearly thirty years later, Dr. Harris and his wife found that much had changed. Tuberculosis had virtually vanished. In 1965, without fully consulting the Dogrib, the federal government decided to move the entire community to the mainland, establishing a medical centre (staffed by nurses) and a school at

Edzo. Yellowknife, sixty miles away, was now the capital of the Northwest Territories and had become the the centre of medical specialist activity. Since Yellowknife was accessible from Edzo by means of the all-weather Mackenzie Highway, the old hospital at Rae had been closed.

As a result of the inspection, our school in Yellowknife was approved by the Canadian Medical Association in June 1981. Shortly thereafter, it was approved as a facility under JCAHPO. This meant that students would take the examinations and be marked by the central organization in competition with students from other parts of Canada and the U.S. This applied to all three levels of competence: assistant, technician and technologist.

This had another benefit, too, in that all staff had to constantly upgrade their reading. The library was improved and Dick Bryan, Jack Clarke and Jeff Oxler were all upgraded to technologists. The first two students to graduate from the Ophthalmic Medical Assistant Training Program did so in 1982. They were two young women from Yellowknife. One young man who had started the course left during his training because he wanted to have time to pursue music, but he discovered the mistake and rejoined the program in time to complete it with the second class. He found ophthalmology and music were quite compatible.

There was a beneficial side effect of this graduation, in that it was now possible to show that students trained entirely in the North could compete on an examination level with those in programs based in hospitals and clinics with facilities greater than those possessed at the Stanton Hospital. The news spread so that applicants—including both Indian and Inuit—came from smaller settlements as far away as Frobisher Bay. The initial scepticism of the university community also passed, and it became possible to have visiting specialists bring their expertise to all the staff. Similarly, our small classes could travel to southern centres where advanced new equipment had been installed, so they could be familiar with procedures carried out by these new techniques should they be discussed in either the written or oral examinations.

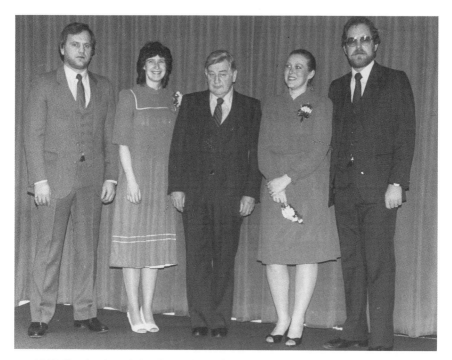

1982 Graduation of the Ophthalmic Medical Assistant Program. Left to right: Dick Bryan, Leslie Bromley, Dr. Graham Gillan, Wendy Brazeau, and Jack Clarke.

Another benefit was that when I went on holiday it was necessary to employ a locum ophthalmologist. Some of our southern colleagues had never seen the North, and were happy to cover for me especially in the summer, when Yellowknife was both beautiful and warm. Some were anxious to visit the settlements and replace me on High Arctic tours. This was particularly true of Col. Forgie and Dr. Bhadresa from Red Deer, who each made multiple trips. Colonel Forgie on his return to Ottawa arranged through a fund subscribed to by the military police for a biomicroscope (slit lamp) to be installed in the Cambridge Bay nursing station.

In all, six students graduated before I retired in 1985. Classes were kept small because the students were to be incorporated into the staff which would eventually supply the whole Northwest Territories, not merely the Mackenzie District of half a million square miles originally serviced. Not more than two could be so absorbed. Because the teaching was financed by the government, we were not able to entertain the application of others, although they were received from as far away as Halifax, Nova Scotia and even Ghana, Africa.

One of the best compliments was an enquiry from some ophthalmologists in Toronto interested in having a similar type of service for northern Ontario. It was also rewarding to hear that a similar training program was set up in Halifax.

My contract with the Stanton Hospital allowed me to attend two congresses a year, and after three years' service that was increased to three annually. This allowed me to keep up with current advances.

It was interesting to compare my medical findings in the western Arctic to those that I had encountered in the Baffin or eastern Arctic zone twenty years before. The myopia among young Inuit was still high, but the phlyctenulosis so prominent in 1965 had almost vanished. An average of about two cases (usually mild) were seen a year, and were found among the Indians and even an occasional Caucasian. Any case in which this appeared was thoroughly checked and followed up by the Department of Health.

The Department of Communicable Disease in Edmonton reported there had been no death from tuberculosis for many years, and most cases being monitored were reactivations of old disease. Now that steroid drops and ointment were readily available the phlycten melted rapidly, and the photophobia lasted only a few days. But it had been a long, hard struggle championed, as I came to learn, by a medical pioneer, Dr. Peter Bryce.

Dr. Bryce, during his stint as chief medical officer of the federal Department of Health in the early part of this century, had been an outspoken critic of government neglect in respect of the rising death rate from tuberculosis among Indians.

Dr. Bryce had inherited a medical mess induced by the toxic mixture of enthusiasm and ignorance. There was apparently no deliberate genocide—only, as we can see in retrospect, wrong priorities. Educate, Christianize, and absorb the Indian into the white society were the pillars of the official policies at that time.

Horrified by statistics coming over his Ottawa desk showing high death rates among Indians attending schools in the North, Dr. Bryce went to inspect the situation for himself. Hampered in many cases by the incompleteness of residential school records, he found that the mortality in these institutions far exceeded the eight per cent his figures had shown.

He also found the rule "no child suffering from scofula or any form of tuberculosis shall be admitted to residence" was not being adhered to. Acute cases were excluded but chronic cases were allowed; otherwise, as one official stated, there would be no scholars.

Dr. Bryce's report of June 19, 1907 records that, of 1,537 scholars reported on, twenty-five per cent were dead. One institution where absolutely accurate records were kept showed that sixty-nine per cent of ex-pupils were dead, almost invariably the diagnosis being tuberculosis.

Dr. Bryce recommended that school residences come under his control and be used as sanitoria. This touched off great opposition from the educational branches of the church-run schools of the time.

While Dr. Bryce's whistle became shriller to draw politicians' attention, the vociferous protests of educators continued until his retirement in 1921. Dr. Bryce was able to have the last word, which shook Ottawa, with the publication of *The Story of a National Crime*.[7]

Now the residential schools are gone and medical care is taken out of the hands of the Department of Mines and Resources (Indian Affairs) and transferred to the national Department of Health and Welfare. Dr. Bryce, who died in 1932, never knew that his successor, Colonel Stone, had the 1936 budget of $50,000 to treat tuberculosis in Indians raised to $4.2 million in 1946.

At that time, 990 Indians were being treated in sanitoria across the country, one of those being the Charles Camsell Hospital in Edmonton. New drugs had entered the scene and a new attitude had come during the war: the red and white men had fought together and had discovered that they were both human, with equally red blood. With these measures, tuberculosis had dropped from first killer in 1952 to eighth place in 1954, and has now decreased to an insignificant level.

Though maps of the nineteenth century show in the Arctic area a section inhabited by Yellowknives, it is remarkable that no one identified themselves as such during the seven years I worked in the area. What had happened to this group? I wrote to Dr. Emoke Szathmary, associate professor of anthropology at McMaster University, who was working on glucose intolerance in the Dogrib people[8] when we were in Yellowknife. She believed the Yellowknives were really Chipewyan, who had found copper from which they were able to make their knives.

Several factors may have contributed to their loss of identity. Reverend Ray Price, for several years a minister in Yellowknife, had recorded the story of early struggles between the Yellowknives and the Dogrib for control of the area north of Great Slave Lake, long claimed by the Dogrib as their fishing preserve, and the final defeat and virtual removal of the Yellowknives from that territory.[9]

Disease took a severe toll. Not only were new diseases such as tuberculosis introduced to the North by white prospectors, but in 1928 an influenza epidemic killed one-sixth of the Dene.[10] It is possible that the remainder were reabsorbed into the parent Chipewyan tribal area.

The influx of the white man was most heavy in the Dogrib area, where gold had been found, and this formed the nucleus of the Caucasian enclave of Yellowknife. Into this area came Dr. Stanton, who formed the first two hospitals bearing his name in the rapidly growing community. This growth was consolidated in 1968 with the transfer of the government centre from Fort Smith to Yellowknife. By the time I first went to work at the Stanton Yellowknife Hospital (the third so named) in 1978, the population had increased to 11,000.

I had heard much of Dr. Oliver Stanton, a legendary figure of the early days of Yellowknife, and every day for more than six years I passed his picture in the hospital. Dr. Stanton was the first, and for many years the only, doctor in the region. He performed the functions of physician, surgeon, radiologist, coroner, hospital administrator and medical officer of health over a vast area.

But there had to be more information on this man who had become a legend. To find it, I approached his friends, many of whom still live in Yellowknife. I started with Jake Woolgar.

As a prospector, Jake had learned to fly in 1935. He first went to Goldfields, Saskatchewan but found that in spite of its name there were no nuggets there. He turned his de Havilland Dragon toward Yellowknife, where gold had really been found. There he was able to get to work. Negus and Con Mine were just starting, with new men coming daily.

There was great excitement in 1937 when two Norseman planes arrived bringing Dr. Oliver Stanton and his vivacious red-haired wife Ruth. They were real assets to the community, both professionally and socially. Though there were 400 men on the little rocky promontory on Great Slave Lake, there were only six women. Besides, the company had provided the Stantons with a home with running water, as well as a six-bed hospital. Ruth, who was a nurse and helped her husband in the hospital, became a social hit with those who were invited for a meal, especially in winter, as it often included a warm bath.

Although Con Mine had taken the initiative in his recruitment, the doctor's services were available, and widely sought, in the large area being explored around Yellowknife. Before Dr. Stanton arrived, the nearest doctor had been at Fort Resolution, across the lake. The medical needs of the miners, prospectors and traders on the north side of the lake were supplied by a first-aid man, Bob Bird.

There were no roads in the area, so many of Stanton's calls made use of Jake's plane. Jake and the doctor travelled to Thompson-Lundmark Mine, seventy miles away, and to injured trappers or prospectors in remote cabins. They travelled to Detah, the Dene village across the bay from Yellowknife. Understanding and friendship developed between the two. "I was the doctor's doctor," says Jake.

When Ollie Stanton was exhausted with his calls, which he had to make on foot at any time of the day or night, Jake would whisk him away in the plane to the Barrens where he could relax while Jake was prospecting.

At the outbreak of the war in 1939 Jake, as a trained pilot, was accepted into the air force and served overseas, partly in the Sicily campaign. Dr. Stanton's application to serve was blocked by the government, since his work in the North was considered an essential service. The mines continued to operate at a maintenance level, returning to full production when the war was over. Jake came back too, and married. Madeleine (Didi) Woolgar and Ruth Stanton became close friends, as both were artists.

Jake remembers being concerned that his friend Ollie was not warmly enough clothed for winter, and once gave him a coat made from a red Hudson's Bay blanket. "You could always tell where the doctor was when he wore that coat," Jake recalls.

Barbara Bromley, who had taken her B.Sc. in nursing before she arrived in Yellowknife in 1948, also remembers the coat. "He really needed it. It was definitely colder in wintertime then, minus fifty or sixty degrees Fahrenheit," she told me.

Barbara gave what time she could in the Red Cross hospital which replaced the mine hospital that year. She remembers Dr. Stanton as gentle in voice and touch. He delivered all her children. She recalls being impressed with his constant concern for his patients. Stanton also took time to be active in the formation of the first Anglican church in Yellowknife, recalls Barbara, and he was so popular that when he ran in the municipal election in 1949 he topped the polls.

Arnold Smith, another long-time Yellowknifer, came to work for the Negus mine in 1939, and continued until its closure in 1952. He recalled the buildings of the era and showed me the first hospital, near the lake, with its windows boarded up. He also showed me the Stanton residence. Together we traced the growth of the community.

Ex-Commissioner John Parker and his wife Helen remember Stanton when they arrived in 1955. Helen was then a social worker, and Ollie took a personal interest in her cases. He was especially concerned with child abuse and neglect.

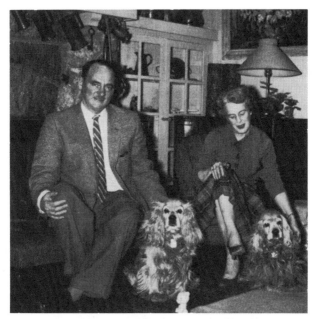

Dr. Oliver Lawson Stanton and his wife.

John McNiven, now a lawyer in Calgary, came to Yellow-knife in 1940. His father, manager at the Negus mine, had arrived two years earlier, but waited until medical services were in place before bringing up his family. John remembers going to school and passing Dr. Stanton's house where his big St. Bernard dog, Monty, would pounce out to play. Stanton knew each child by name and always took time to talk to each one.

John also remembers the fire at the Negus bunkhouse in 1943. When the alarm sounded John, 13, ran toward the fire but Dr. Stanton, bag in hand, passed him on the mile-long run to the blaze. The fire was out of control. The water pipes from the lake were wrapped in muskeg as insulation, and enclosed in a wooden frame. This too was ablaze and it was some time before enough water was available to douse the flames. Three miners perished that night—tragic illustration of the hazards of northern living.

Stanton graduated in 1929 from the University of Toronto, in the era before the explosion of scientific medicine and wonder drugs. The sulphas had been introduced, and penicillin became available during World War II, but Ollie had other therapeutic agents which science has difficulty assessing. Stanton could also inspire faith, which is a major component of healing. Modern medicine with its gadgetry can keep the body alive but it takes faith, and the optimism it produces, to make one live.

Ruth Stanton, in a letter in 1987, gave me another secret of his success—love. She said: "Ollie worked himself out, carried the load too long, but he really loved the place and people."

Does love have healing power? Science has always doubted anything it could not measure, but we now have statistics from insurance companies that affection in the home reduces accidents and keeps people alive five years longer. Dr. Bernie Siegal, who compiled the results, believes that love is the most powerful known stimulant to the immune system, and produces measurable biological results in a person.[11]

Dr. Oliver Lawson Stanton was a good doctor. Although I never met him, I know because his patients say so. They are the real judges. Yellowknifers returned his affection. At the July 1 party before he left the community, they gathered to honour him. All his "babies" wore "I am a Stanton baby" button in their lapels. There were a lot of them. And many of them still remember Yellowknife's first doctor. Oliver Stanton retired to Salt Spring Island, British Columbia in 1960 and died there ten years later, but the hospital that bears his name is a fitting monument.

The Indians we served in Hay River at the H. H. Williams Memorial Hospital were mainly Slavey and Cree, and at the Fort Smith Health Centre there were more Cree. This latter group had moved into Denendeh from their usual habitat further south to escape the smallpox ravaging the plains. Other Indian tribes of the Mackenzie Valley—the Hareskin and Loucheux—fell within the purview of the Inuvik Hospital further north, although some no doubt visited Yellowknife for business with the government or for work.

Though much has been learned about the Indian tribes, there is much that still needs to be untangled, and it is possible that a study of one of the eye diseases commonly found in the

North may help to untangle this. It was soon clear after my arrival in Yellowknife that there was a disproportionately high incidence of anterior uveitis (inflammation of the iris and ciliary body) occurring in Indian populations. Dr. Elizabeth Cass had noticed this, but had attributed much of it to the tuberculosis prevalent at the time.[12] By now tuberculosis was no longer a feature of northern medicine, but still the cases continued.

As many of these cases also had arthritis of various joints, I had a discussion with Dr. Michael Igoe, the internist at Stanton Hospital.[13] He referred me to research which was coming to the fore in genetics. Workers in the field of haematology had been finding in white blood cells, or leucocytes, factors which made every person as distinct as their fingerprints. This had been given the name of Human Leucocyte Antigen (HLA) and the various factors were assigned letters and numbers. The occurrence of certain of these factors in specific diseases was being carefully studied, and soon the presence of HLA B27 was noticed in patients suffering from eye and joint disease similar to what we were finding.

Tests, especially those produced by recent research, were technically beyond the capacity of an ordinary hospital laboratory such as the one at Stanton Hospital. They were available in Edmonton, 600 air miles south, but not on a daily basis. This meant a great deal of synchronisation between the laboratories, and transportation. The tests were expensive and climate and time were of the essence, so the white blood cells could be in a state in which a valid reading could be given.

To my wife, Annelise, fell a great deal of the arranging as coordinator of the laboratory. To meet plane schedules, samples had to be drawn at certain times and a courier dispatched to transport specimens to the Alberta Provincial Laboratory in Edmonton on arrival. In spite of our best efforts, some samples were unsuitable, or at best equivocal, as often the patient had returned home hundreds of miles away before the blood's unsuitability could be reported to the hospital.

In spite of the difficulties it was soon apparent that the incidence of people of the surrounding tribes carrying the HLA B27 factor in their blood was higher than the national average of six per cent. High percentages of this factor were also being found in the blood of Indians in other regions: the Haida on the British Columbia Coast had 50 per cent; the Navajo cousins of our Dogrib people had 25 per cent and the Pima Indians 18 per cent. The Greenland Inuit were also recorded to have 18 per cent.

Dr. Michael Igoe was able to obtain a grant for a survey of the incidence of HLA B27 in the Dogrib population in their largest community, Rae-Edzo. The result showed 40 per cent carried the troublesome factor.[14] As this genetic marker is present at birth and carried through life, our cases of recurrent uveitis and arthritis could only be treated symptomatically, not cured.

Another problem requiring considerable investigation was that of the night blindness occurring in young as well as older people in the Dogrib community of Rae-Edzo. The public health nurse, Sister Louise Brosseau, and a social worker reported the matter to us, and the problem was identified as Retinitis Punctata Albescens, a disease with the same symptoms as Retinitis Pigmentosa, but where the deposits on the retina are white instead of black. There is much disability associated with the disease—virtual blindness out of doors during the long, dark winter months. I contacted the Canadian National Institute for the Blind to help in training the affected to become more independent. Unfortunately, when I contacted the Alberta provincial headquarters in Edmonton, I found there was no budget for the Northwest Territories. Apparently, when the Provincial Divisions were formed, there had been no request from the North, and so it was left out. On a visit to Edmonton, I strongly protested this, saying that I was sure, as one who had known Colonel Baker, that he wanted the whole country serviced. After application to the Toronto headquarters, supervision for the whole Northwest Territories was added to the Alberta Division, whose card now carries the title, "The Canadian National Institute for the Blind, Alberta–N.W.T. Division." The current area representative in Yellowknife is Lydia Bardak, who is continuing the care for the needs of her large terrritory.

The retinal disease was soon identified as being an autosomal recessive disorder. In a society where hunting and trapping is still a way of life, this disease (in which the main feature is night blindness) imperilled the next generation. What made the hazard more difficult to control was that carriers had been identified in every family group of the tribe, so any intermarriage would certainly increase the incidence of cases.

Because of the long winter nights, with only about two hours of daylight in December, the males were not able to reach any traplines. The defect also made it virtually impossible for the afflicted to obtain work with government departments such as heavy-duty operators on snowplows, in the winter months. In the summer, with the virtual absence of darkness, working was feasible as long as vision remained good enough. As this condition is considered to be a version of Retinitis Pigmentosa, where there is no effective treatment, the prospect remains bleak.

There being no therapy for the condition, education of the entire tribe became essential. With the help of the incumbent priest and Sister Louise Brosseau, a Grey Nun nurse, a meeting was arranged. Representatives of the CNIB and the department of Social Services, on whom most of the rehabilitation would fall, were happy to meet with the mothers of affected children. I presented the main features of the disease. Dr. W. G. Pearce, who had worked with me in Newfoundland and was now a professor at the University of Alberta, was able to use the family trees prepared by Sister Louise to show the genetic transmission.

A separate meeting was later held with the chief and some elders, with the priest acting as interpreter. The impact of the disease on the tribe was of great concern to them. It was emphasized that intertribal marriage should be actively discouraged, and that spouses should be sought from nearby tribes. I knew some Navajo from Arizona had visited their cousins in the North and had been able to understand each other's dialect, though the northern and southern branches had separated centuries before. I wondered if there would be benefit by relinking the two branches by marriage.

The CNIB representatives who continue to monitor the children will no doubt try to reinforce the message. An effort is being made to identify the carriers. New frontiers in genetic engineering are opening which may someday help correct defects, but whether they will be accepted by the tribe remains doubtful. The solution must rest with the tribe itself.

While some diseases of the eye are more commonly found among the indigenous inhabitant, there was a marked scarcity of conditions which I had found among my patients in Toronto and Newfoundland. Disease of the retinal arteries, associated with hypertension, arteriosclerosis and diabetes were rarely seen among the Inuit. Diabetes was at one time considered to be absent in this group, and rare in the Indian.

That this is slowly changing was stressed in several papers presented at the Sixth International Symposium of Circumpolar Health[15] held in Anchorage, Alaska in May 1984. There seemed to be consensus among those who had studied the general health and fitness in northern Canada, Alaska, and Siberia that with the virtual abandonment of the nomadic way of life, with its great exercise component, and with the dependence on imported southern food, the incidence of incipient diabetes had increased. The Indians had now shown several cases of diabetic retinopathy, requiring laser treatment. Figures were also presented showing the increase in body mass, among males particularly, between the years 1971 and 1981.

The indigenous group most studied relative to change in life-style and diet are the Pima Indians of Arizona. In them the reduction of physical activity and the consumption of "white man's food" produced a marked increase in diabetes. With the gathering of nomadic hunters into settlements in the North, and the greater use of imported food, the picture may be repeated. Unless some prevention or treatment can be found for diabetes, retinal artery disease may increase in the North.

With the service running well, it was time for me to step aside. Travelling and the long, hard winters made me feel in need of a change. The University of Alberta in Edmonton, which was our main referral centre, had an ophthalmologist whom they recommended and who was interested in the North and the type of scheme developed to service remote regions. At the end of July 1985, I was able to hand everything over to Dr. Leonard Smith, and Annelise and I drove south.

On the long road south there was plenty of time to assess what had been accomplished during the seven years we had spent working in Yellowknife. While I was looking forward to the next phase of life, my wife had so enjoyed her stay that she was loath to leave.

Nevertheless, there was a sense of satisfaction that we had both left our imprint on medical care north of the sixtieth parallel, as we waved goodbye to the three-legged bear which guarded that line.

Annelise had standardized the three hospital laboratories at Yellowknife, Hay River and Fort Smith to the new metric system imposed by the federal government. Improvement had been made to the equipment and more tests introduced. One great difficulty remained in the nursing stations which were still under federal control, and that was in the bacteriological identification of organisms. Swabs taken during the cold months of the year were invariably negative by the time they reached the laboratory in Yellowknife. Frequently given to the pilot to deliver at the hospital, they were often too cold or too old to be of value. By the use of a new method using ISOCULTS,[16] the nurse could have helpful results quickly. The medium was made up in a selective way, encouraging the growth of some organisms and inhibiting others, thereby making visual diagnosis possible by colour changes. Thus, in forty-eight hours, the nurses could have some idea of which group of organisms was creating the pathology, and which antibiotic, if any, would be most helpful. Otherwise, some of these expensive drugs would be wasted treating virus conditions which they would not benefit.

The result of her experience in the North was shared in three scientific papers.[17] Interestingly enough, it was the Health Services in Alaska that sensed the value of this methodology, as they too were dealing with small scattered communities with the same problems of climate and transportation as prevailed in the Northwest Territories.

I, too, was able to look back with some pleasure. There was now an eye service which gave access to care to each of the people in the scattered Land of the Midnight Sun, since each community was visited at least once a year by the team, and the larger places several times annually. There was also a good filing system in the eye clinic in Yellowknife, with notes on each eye patient visiting Yellowknife or the nursing station clinics. This method of duplicate charts made follow-up easy.

The Ophthalmic Medical Assistant Training Program had given an opportunity for the people in the North to train and compete with those training in the large centres, and to succeed.

Arctic College, which operated on a similar concept, would later expand to further this equalizing force. During my fifty years as a physician (over forty of these spent in Canada as an ophthalmologist) it has been my privilege to see tremendous strides not only in my own specialty, but also in education. As public health is a larger concept than can be handled by physicians only, so education is a project which embraces more than professional educators; it affects us all. As education goes, so goes the country.

No closer bond can occur than between ophthalmologists and teachers. Almost all children with reading difficulties have their eyes blamed for their problems. Parents are the last to accept the fact that seeing and comprehension are two different faculties.

In the Northwest Territories, distances were great and the population small, making the impact of the southern world hard to absorb. In the sixties, there was a rise of native consciousness, as educated Indian and Inuit began to challenge the paternalism of the federal government. The old order in the North was changing; development of resources was beginning to occur. If the people of the North were to derive their rightful share of employment, they must have the technical skills.

This first took shape in 1968, when a heavy equipment course was commenced at Fox Hole, twenty-two miles from Fort Smith. In 1969, this facility was moved to Fort Smith and named the Adult Vocational Training Centre (AVTC). This was not surprising, as there are probably more caterpillar tractors and road graders per capita in the Northwest Territories than in any other place in North America. The AVTC quickly became a success. In 1981, it was granted college status and its name changed to Thebacha College.

In 1982, the principal of Thebacha College visited the eye clinic. He wanted no examination; his eyes were fine. It was clear that though the bulk of the budget and operation of the school for ophthalmic technicians came through medical channels, the Department of Education was using it as a pilot project.

As the Department of Health started to take over the administration of hospital and nursing stations from the federal Department of Health and Welfare, the travel area of technicians increased. Pathology found was reported to the ophthalmologist responsible for each section.

By 1990, Thebacha College was no longer the only point of advanced education in the North, for it was called the Thebacha Campus of the Arctic College, one of six operated by that body. From its head office in Yellowknife, Arctic College also operated the Aurora Campus in Inuvik, Nunatta Campus in Frobisher Bay, Keewatin Campus in Rankin Inlet, Kitikmeot Campus in Cambridge Bay, and a campus in Yellowknife. Around each of the campuses are Learning Centres, forty in all, to raise standards at the local level.

As Canada starts to run short of resources, it will turn North again. Multinational corporations have in the past brought workers from the south because they claimed there are not enough people trained in modern skills. Arctic College now says it has been producing a pool of personnel trained in using maintenance equipment for the ice roads, computer-trained personnel for the mines, health and nursing assistants for clinics, and secretarial staff for the offices. These graduates are all North-friendly—knowing how to handle the climatic extremes of their territory, they are not alien spirits in an unforgiving land.

Thus, as we drove south, it was with an element of satisfaction. The time between the regular retirement age and seventy had not been frittered away in wasteful idleness. We both felt that we had left something of ourselves in the North which contributed to its betterment. We too had learned and shared many of the problems faced by other Arctic dwellers, which made us in many ways closer to our neighbours in Greenland, Siberia, northern Finland and Scandinavia, than to the 3,000-mile-distant Ottawa bureaucrats.

Retirement means different things to different people. For some, it means golf, sailing, or a life of idleness. For me, it meant a set of new tires for another run, for there was still much to do and to see.

Some years before, we had purchased a beautiful chalet-style home in the idyllic setting of the foothills of the Rockies at Canmore, Alberta, but, when 1985 came, some problems arose. While still fit enough to enjoy the outdoors, both my wife and I found ourselves too mentally restless; we wanted to do university courses and find fulfilling volunteer occupations. These were more likely to be found in a city such as Calgary, so we moved there.

This gave ready access to the continuing education courses in anthropology and history, as well as the wonderful Arctic Institute library at the University of Calgary. This is reported to have the best sources of information on the North in the Americas.

An opportunity arose in 1986 to go to China with a special group of missionaries' "children" who had been born in that country. It was designed to visit places associated with our youth. It gave me an opportunity to check on what had happened to the Christian Church in the land in which my parents had spent so much time, and in which my father is buried. My mother returned there, and was interned during World War II. Fortunately, she survived, though she was seventy years of age when released. I was delighted to find that the task my parents and other missionaries had tried to accomplish had indeed borne fruit. Christians who had been estimated as numbering about one million in 1949 were now reported to be about forty million and growing. As my children had not had a chance to know their grandparents, I recorded for them, and others interested in church growth, the story of my mother's arrival in

Shanghai in 1901, just after the Boxer rising, to the time of my return eighty-five years later, in a book called *The Seed Must Grow*.

The year, 1987, was eventful in that I was honoured, along with other colleagues, by the Canadian Ophthalmological Society with a special award which was given "in appreciation of outstanding contribution to medical eye care in Canada" at the fiftieth anniversary of its founding. This recognition by peers is a very precious possession, and the medal and framed citation are proudly displayed in our living room.

It is natural, as the years pass that we examine and assess our relationships. One built-in product of life is pain. This is not all bad; it can be very productive: we are all the product of our mothers' pain.

It is probable that there would not have been a project in Newfoundland in 1964 if there had been no trauma of separation and loneliness in 1962. While rest is necessary in the treatment of fractured bones, broken relationships are usually rendered less severe by work intense enough to give no time for brooding: hence many workaholics.

On the steeper trails of the mountain of life which we had now entered, we might at times have to use a lower gear, but neither of us want to go into park. We had fallen in love with the life and the people of the North, into so many of whose eyes I had looked. Now I wanted to paint word pictures of that life for those who have not had the privilege.

Time is a great healer, and the communication with the family is restored stronger than ever: they love Annelise and she reciprocates. Visiting in the United States, where they are located, is limited by distance, but my monthly telephone bill tells me exactly how much quality time is spent on a one-to-one basis with each. The family increased by one in 1990 when a great grandson was born. To hold such a one in my arms diverts the vision from the past to the future. What more can a man want?

Appendix A

CNIB Sight Defect Detection Surveys: 1967-70

Date	Place	Total Tested	Referred for Examination
October 1967	Labrador City	522	84
	Wabush	273	60
March/September 1968	Mount Pearl	808	82
May 1968	Corner Brook	1803	189
October 1968	Appleton, Benton, Gander, Glenwood	795	68
February/March 1969	Bishops Falls	335	26
	Botwood	296	32
	Buchans	220	35
	Buchans Junction	29	1
	Grand Falls	544	71
	Millertown	23	1
	Peterview	70	12
	Windsor	543	78
June 1969	Happy Valley	473	82
	Northwest River	99	10
May 1969	Badger[1]	75	11
September 1969	Baie Verte	220	36
	Brent's Cove	53	8
	Coachman's Cove	11	-
	Fleur-de-Lys	17	3
	Harbour Round	-	-
	LaScie	87	14
	Purbeck's Cove	4	1
	Round Harbour	-	-
	Shoe Cove	17	1
	Tilt Cove	8	1
	Westport	1	1
October 1969	Gander[2]	180	21
February/March 1970	*Burin Peninsula*		
	Burin[3]	342	88
	Fortune	139	27
	Grand Bank	185	33
	Lamaline	55	6
	Lawn	124	18
	Marystown[4]	355	76
	St. Lawrence	171	35

April 1970	Badger	107	25
	Springdale		
	Beachside	22	8
	Card's Harbour	7	1
	Gullbridge Mines	15	5
	Harry's Harbour	17	1
	Jackson's Cove	15	5
	Jim's Cove	9	1
	King's Point	44	15
	Little Bay	38	14
	Pilley's Island	23	3
	Rattling Brook	13	1
	Roberts Arm	111	22
	St. Patricks	16	3
	South Brook	67	15
	Springdale	263	52
	Triton	36	6
July 1970	Lamaline[1]	50	1
	Totals:	9730	1389

1 Follow-up PHN.

2 Follow-up Lionettes

3 *Including*: Big Salmonier, Black Duck Cove, Bull's Cove, Burin Bay Arm, Collin's Cove, Epworth, Fox Cove, Harfett, Lewin's Cove, Little Salmonier, Mortier, Path End, Paul's Hill, Port au Bras, Salt Pond, and Ship Cove.

4 *Including*: Creston North, Creston South, Little Bay, Marystown North, and Marystown South.

Appendix B

CNIB SIGHT DEFECT DETECTION SURVEYS BY YEAR

DATE	TOTAL TESTED	REFERRED FOR EXAMINATION
1967	795	144
1968	3406	339
1969	3305	445
1970	2224	461
Total	9730	1389

Appendix C

CNIB Sight Defect Detection Surveys by District

Date	Place	Total Tested		Referred for Examination	
	East				
1968	Mount Pearl	808		82	
1970	Burin Peninsula	1371		283	
	Lamaline[1]	50		1	
			2229		366
	Central				
1968	Gander	795		68	
1969	Badger[2]	75		11	
	Baie Verte	418		65	
	Bishops Falls	335		26	
	Botwood	366		44	
	Buchans	272		37	
	Gander[1]	180		21	
	Grand Falls	544		71	
	Windsor	543		78	
1970	Badger	107		25	
	Springdale	696		152	
			4331		598
	West				
1967	Labrador City	522		84	
	Wabush	273		60	
1968	Corner Brook	1803		189	
1969	Happy Valley	473		82	
	Northwest River	99		10	
			3170		425

1 Follow-up.
2 Follow-up PHN.

Appendix D | Canada's Northland is Challenging You*

C ANADA HAS TWO FACES—the sophisticated face of the provinces and the unadorned rugged face of the North. The southern provincial area is well-developed by roads, rails, canals and competing airlines. It is possible to pass over all the ten provinces by the fastest possible jet, in record time. In the cities larger and larger buildings are developed and as if there is no room for all the people to keep their feet on the ground, they live and work in increasing numbers elevated in layer upon layer, storey upon storey.

Geography

In contrast to all this provincial development and the rivalry as to who can have the biggest and best, is the Northwest Territory administered by the federal government. Here is an area of 1.5 million square miles with a population density of approximately one person for every four square miles. This population, besides being thin, is not evenly spaced. A look at the map of Canada suggests to the doctor a picture of the upper jaw. Eight of Canada's ten provinces and the western Arctic, although honeycombed by lakes and dotted by islands, represent a large, continuous land mass. On the eastern side is a very large inlet, composed of Hudson and James Bays which appear like the maxillary sinus. Two Canadian provinces, Prince Edward Island and Newfoundland (plus the eastern Arctic), are so broken as to represent teeth on this jaw, which is arranged to snap on and engulf the Polar Sea. Some of the rugged area in the region of the eastern part of Baffin Land, with glacial peaks rising up to

* Reprinted from *Among the Deep Sea Fishers* (International Grenfell Association), Vol. 64, No. 2, July 1966, pp. 41-45.

8,000 feet straight out of deep fiords, enhances the idea of the toothlike picture on the map.

It will, therefore, be quite obvious to the reader that while the idea of equal medical care for all is something for which we should constantly strive, the element of *geography* makes the attainment of this ideal more difficult and in some cases almost impossible. While on the flatter land of the western Arctic, road transportation is possible, this form of transportation is virtually impossible in the eastern Arctic. Here in the summer boats busily supply the various ports. There has to be careful planning ahead so that all the items which are likely to be needed for the next ten or eleven months are ordered so that they can be brought in on the sea lift. In the wintertime, things can be delivered by plane, but this of course is expensive. The period of break-up in the early summer and freeze-up in the fall are times which are most critical. In these periods, contact by water and by air are very difficult and quite often impossible. Units of medical personnel, therefore, whether lay dispenser, medical orderly, registered nurse or doctor, have periods of isolation when often they have to rely on their own judgment and on help given by radio. For this reason it cannot be too strongly emphasized that nursing personnel must be of the highest quality.

Due to transportation difficulties, facilities are used to the maximum. The plane taking the writer in to the Grenfell Mission, for example, was bringing out two very sick people. One was a woman with post-partum haemorrhage, who had arrived some days before at the station, pulseless. With the use of supportive care and blood expanders, it was possible to keep her alive during three days of storm, and then send her to hospital headquarters at St. Anthony, Newfoundland, for further help.

The second case was one of severe pneumonia which developed an empyema. By the use of antibiotics, oxygen and careful nursing, this case was kept going until the storm abated sufficiently to allow the plane to transport him to St. Anthony. The empyema was so gross that the pleural cavity could be evacuated only a little at a time. The case finally recovered.

Both these cases were cared for by the nurse in charge of the nursing station. This nurse was also running a small hospital of eleven beds, an obstetrical service, well-baby clinic and general care of the surrounding community. There is radio-telephone contact with the main hospital at St. Anthony three times a day. This provided consultation with, and guidance from, the doctors based there, until her patients were transferred to that hospital.

It is a great pity that too often Canadian-trained nurses do not rise to the standards necessary to this type of isolated practice. While Canadian nurses from various centres work in the hospitals of the Northwest Territory, quite a number of the nurses in isolated stations are from Australia or Europe.

Most of our Canadian nursing schools are located in and slanted to the needs of the large centres. That there are areas where doctors are few or inaccessible, even in the provinces, is ignored. Nurses trained in midwifery are essential for the more isolated and northern communities.

Too often Canadian-trained doctors are apt to stick to the cities and it has been found difficult to recruit the medical personnel for more rugged work in the northland. It was the experience of the writer that in a hospital in the eastern Arctic, of three medical officers in residence, two were from Britain and one (working on the Dew Line sites) was from India.

Economics

While the foregoing has dealt mainly with the challenge of geography, there is also the challenge of *economics*. In order to service as many people as possible, the federal government has equipped and runs a ship called the *C. D. Howe*, which plies between Montreal and most, if not all, of the settlements in the eastern Arctic easily reached by boat. This ship visits ports on the way northward, crossing the Arctic circle and visiting the most northerly island (Ellesmere). Then, it gradually works its way down by another route and so out through Hudson Strait to the Labrador Sea and back up the St. Lawrence before the freeze-up commences. While this is an expensive trip, it is about the only feasible way of covering the eastern Arctic. Once the freeze has set in, medical supplies and personnel must be brought in by air. The round-trip fare from Montreal to Frobisher Bay, approximately 1,650 miles north of Montreal, is $250. This means that if four patients have to be sent to hospital in Montreal, the minimum cost for transportation is $1,000. Also, for those patients there is the cost of medical care and of boarding out until transportation home is available; all this has to be paid for by the government until a plane can be found or the patient is considered fit enough to return north. As there are approximately three or four scheduled flights a week to Frobisher Bay and points further north, there are obviously gaps in the timing and should a severe emergency arise that requires urgent evacuation to a main centre, then a special plane must be chartered at a cost of approximately $3,500–$4,000.

While the cost of medical care may seem very great, the cost of *not* giving adequate medical care may be even greater. Thus, patients who are disabled or partially disabled may be a liability to the public purse for many years. Social assistance is administered mainly through the Department of Northern Affairs and Natural Resources, but perhaps more could be done to develop the Eskimo's natural inventiveness. The Eskimo who inhabits the Northland is very hardy and a natural mechanic. It sometimes happens that if some of the machinery made of steel, which can become very brittle in the cold, breaks under stress, and parts have to be sent by air from the nearest large centre, a great deal of time is consumed. The local authority must sanction this purchase, then the headquarters, and so on down the line. By the time the part has been returned, the tractor or other motorized vehicle may be running with a spare part made by the Eskimo out of ivory! The biggest contribution that can be made to the Eskimo is to help him develop himself. Often this can only be done through preventive medicine and this will be discussed later.

It would be very wrong to give the impression that economics in the north represents the payment by the federal government of large sums of money to keep the health of those in the northern areas well maintained. The north also contributes economically to the general weal of Canada. Prospectors have explored and found fabulous metal deposits in the north. One of the newest and possibly richest has been found at Mary River, and a town site is being made several hundred miles north of Frobisher Bay. It is also possible that there are deposits of oil and other natural treasures hidden in this treeless area.

Perhaps in the next twenty-five or fifty years, great wagons or trains, operating on the hover-craft principle will operate down the coast of the eastern Arctic, bringing huge supplies of metal to keep the people in the south in work. Because of the danger to Canada and to the United States of assault over the North Pole, warning posts were established, with the two countries sharing in the expense. This has done much to open up the North, which had been relatively neglected since the early days when pioneers from Europe, especially Britain and France explored the country.

Medical Matters

Having defined some of the problems of geography and economics, it is now necessary for us to look at how some of the problems in *medical matters* are being and can be solved. Firstly, it must be said that while from the purely legal point of view, medicine in Canada is a provincial affair, doctors have always realized that medical need and medical care are not only national but international. The federal government has provided the N.W. Territory under its control with hospitals and nursing stations strategically placed. The staffing of these we have discussed. One of the problems, however, that still remains is how to reach with adequate care those who require a specialist's treatment. While there will always be a few cases requiring immediate transportation facilities, many of those requiring help are on the elective list, and means are being developed to help these more. The Children's Hospital in Montreal is sending to Frobisher Bay one of its residents in paediatrics who will work in this hospital in the north as part of his routine course. Meanwhile, Queen's University in Kingston has a working arrangement with the federal hospital at Moosoonee. The writer of this article visited the Grenfell Mission hospital in St. Anthony, Newfoundland–Labrador, recently, and also the hospital at Frobisher Bay in the eastern Arctic. In the former instance, it was possible to fly into nursing stations of the Grenfell Mission and see cases requiring ophthalmic care. While many adults were seen, it was noted particularly that there were quite a number of children who needed care of refractive problems if they were going to be able to study sufficiently to fill a place in the modern world. At Frobisher Bay, it was possible to review during one month's stay the total school population of the area. There are approximately 900 of the Eskimo community and about 600 others (mainly government servants and families) who form the population of this town.

The hospital at Frobisher Bay is small but well-equipped, and it was possible to do some strabismus surgery on cases which had previously been selected in visits by ophthalmologists on the *C. D. Howe*. This was accomplished only because of the supreme efforts of the medical and nursing staff who are operating at two thirds of the required personnel on establishment. The surgery was also made possible by the introduction of an anaesthetic specialist who flew up to work a concentrated 48-hour stint.

As previously pointed out, in the section on economics, it is much more economical to send in a specialist than to ship out approximately ten patients by air at $250 each for transportation costs only. Development of this type of thing, particularly in the field of ear, nose and throat surgery, would be a tremendous asset. It seems rather stupid from the economic point of view to fly out children for tonsillectomy and for advice on deafness when so much could be done at a local level. A suggested approach would be the production of a flying squad consisting of surgeon, anaesthetist, two nurses (male or female). Cases for surgery could be organized by the local medical staff prior to the arrival of the team. The surgeon could then check the cases pre-operatively, the anaesthetist could check his equipment and schedules could be set up. The nurses could have liaison with their counterparts on the field. Two days of intensive surgery would probably be as much as the hospital could hold. Then the other members of the team could leave, while the specialist stayed on for two or three more days watching for any post-operative complications and seeing cases requiring medical opinion. If much post-operative care by nurses were required, then one or both nurses could stay and return with the surgeon. Concentrated work for a week could do a great deal to break the bottleneck in the present system.

While the medical profession can contribute in this way immediately, a great deal must be done by the administrators of nursing programmes and particularly by the government. While the government has helped to make the North more economically attractive, the Ministry of Health has not done so much as might be expected, in areas such as the provision of better housing for the nurses in the eastern Arctic.

One area of planning on a long-term basis warrants special consideration. The Arctic is essentially "home" to the Eskimo; it follows, therefore, that suitable local personnel should be trained in observation and nursing arts, so that they can work among their own people. Such training schools could form an area of coöperation between the Departments of Northern Affairs and Natural Resources and Health and Welfare. The personnel thus trained could report daily by radio-telephone to describe conditions and receive instructions. These could replace R.C.M.P., Hudson's Bay store managers and others who are now acting as lay dressers.

Much is being done—but much more is necessary, in the Arctic. The Northwest Territory is not a province; it is still under federal care. It is therefore a responsibility, and a challenge to every Canadian.

Appendix E | *The Cornea in Canada's Northland**

MAN'S DEPENDENCE ON his inheritance and his surroundings is the theme of recurrent investigation. This
theme in relation to northern Canada will be pursued in this
article. Although all kinds of eye problems are encountered,
only those characteristic of the area will be stressed.

A number of trips have been made to central and northern
Newfoundland and Labrador since 1964. A month was spent in
Frobisher Bay. Since no visits were made to the western Arctic,
the material refers to the eastern Arctic and sub-Arctic areas
only.

Congenital defects

Congenital defects of the cornea were found infrequently in the
Eskimo children examined. One baby was encountered similar
to the cases described by Speakman and Crawford[1] In Newfoundland, in areas where consanguinity was high, many congenital iris abnormalities have been found, but few corneal
lesions. Embryotoxon has been noted on two occasions.

Phlyctenulosis

This is reportedly the commonest cause of blindness in the
Arctic. On the visit to Frobisher Bay, 271 patients were seen of
whom 189 were of the Eskimo race. Of these, six had active
phlyctenulosis and 41 had scarring of the cornea. Of this latter
group, 25 were considered of phlyctenular origin and 16 of un-
determined cause. Thus, phlyctenulosis was present in active or

* Reprinted from the *Canadian Journal of Ophthalmology*, Vol. 5, No. 2, April 1970,
 pp. 146-51.

TABLE I

PHLYCTENULOSIS

Age: Common in childhood.
Sex: Found equally in male and female.
Location: Occurs at any part of limbus and spreads centrally. Sub-epithelial abscess, which breaks down.
Secondary Infection: Common. May be severe enough to produce perforation.
Etiology: Vitamin deficiency especially 'C.' Sensitization to bacterial protein. 35–85% T.B. found.
Treatment: Medical. Effect of steroids dramatic but transient. Vitamin replacement necessary for permanent cure. Vitamin 'C' I.V. and oral. Desensitization by T.B. protein.[19]

LABRADOR KERATOPATHY

Age: Found in those over 40.
Sex: Very few if any females. Exclusively male disease.
Location: Opacity in interpalpebral fissure, under upper lid clear. Deep to Bowman's membrane.
Secondary Infection: Not commoner than usual. Association with pterygium high.
Etiology: Exposure to weather—low relative humidity and fine ice particles.
Treatment: Effect of steroid nil. Keratoplasty – Lamellar rotation graft.

---

quiescent form in 16.3% of the Eskimo cases seen. This condition is reportedly common also in the Eskimo population in northern Labrador, but it is rare in the non-Eskimo, in Labrador and the island of Newfoundland. Some of the distinguishing points between phlyctenulosis and Labrador keratopathy which will be discussed later are listed in Table I.

Labrador Keratopathy

This has been so well described by Arnold Freedman[2] that only certain points need to be stressed:

(*a*) It occurs only in older age groups, being more severe in patients over 40 years. It is seen very rarely, if ever, in females.
(*b*) It is not associated with photophobia.
(*c*) It is not associated with secondary infection.
(*d*) It is frequently associated with pterygium formation.

Pterygium

This is quite common in Newfoundland especially among fishermen. In a recent random survey in the northern peninsula of that island, the following figures were found:

TABLE II		*Pterygia*
Men over 40 years	39	13
Women over 40 years	55	2
Men under 40 years	16	0
Women under 40 years	39	1
Total Adults	149	
Total Children	144	none

Pterygia are often very large and in long-standing cases may cross the pupil to reduce vision to the guiding level only.

DISCUSSION

Phlyctenulosis: This disease, which was relatively common in the writer's student days over thirty years ago, is now relatively rare in most parts of the world. Nevertheless, its frequency in the Arctic is attested to by the figures given previously by writers such as Reed and Hildes,[3] Farson[4] and others who have visited and worked there. The etiology of phlyctenulosis is still stimulating considerable discussion, but certain factors appear to be important:

1. The condition is associated with infection, but no constant infective agent has been noted in the lesion itself.
2. It has affected people of all colours and racial origins in all parts of the world. It has been noted among the Caucasian races, the Mongolian and Negroid peoples.
3. It has shown some seasonable incidence. After reviewing the European literature Sorsby[5] pointed out that the highest incidence of the condition was in the months of January to May. This does not appear to apply to Africa according to the report of Stein and Freiman.[6] From personal observation it does not seem to apply in the Arctic. This variation in itself is significant.
4. The incidence of the disease has shown a decrease in Europe between 1912 and 1932.
5. The disease is associated with poor nutrition.
6. Phlyctenulosis is associated with a hyper-sensitivity state.
7. The condition responds rapidly to local steroid therapy.

Some points in relation to these factors are important:

1. The frequency of association with tuberculosis is very marked and these two conditions have been found associated in from 35 to 85% of cases in recorded series. Other infections have also been incriminated, e.g. staphylococcus aureus and systemic gonococcal infection.

2. The fact that it affects all races of people in all parts of the world shows probably climatic conditions have very little to do with the condition. Also, the presence or absence of pigment has nothing to do with the development of the phlycten in the eye.

3. It is also very interesting that the seasonal incidence of the condition has varied in different parts of the world. During the period when phlyctenulosis was common in Europe, it was noted that the highest incidence of the disease was between the months of January and May when the sun shone least. In fact, some of the European writers claimed that it was the absence of sunshine that contributed to the production of phlyctenulosis.

During the months of January to May, there was little if any, local production of green vegetables with consequent reduction in vitamin C. In the warmer climates there is no time when no fresh fruit or vegetables are available, whereas in the Arctic there is no season in which fruits and vegetables are produced. (The Eskimo does increase his diet during the summer by gathering and eating berries.) In the two extremes of climate there are no seasonal variations in the incidence of phlyctenulosis.

4. The marked decline in phlyctenulosis in the period 1912–32 introduces an interesting note into our search for the etiology of this condition. In the latter part of the nineteenth century and the beginning of the twentieth century, phlyctenulosis was probably at its height. It is true that there was a lot of tuberculosis at this time, but it is possible that the diseases had one common denominator, rather than that one was the product of the other. The Industrial Revolution took many people from their farms and crowded them in cities where they often ate potatoes, bread, jam and other starchy foods which were cheap and easily acquired. Overcrowding led to an increase in infections of all types.

5. The role of diet is recognized by Duke-Elder[7] who wrote "diet too, should be corrected by cutting down carbohydrates to a minimum, by prescribing a relatively high intake of protein, with an abundance of vitamins, particularly ascorbic acid." Significantly, it was in 1907 that the final link in the chain of evidence was forged by Holst and Frolich[8] showing that vitamin C was the anti-scorbutic agent. With the dissemination of knowledge about this new preparation, the fact that it could not be stored well in the body and that a constant supply was necessary, the attention of people in general was turned to the necessity of having fresh fruit and vegetables in their diet. This, in turn, increased their ability to withstand disease and so simultaneously assisted in the reduction of phlyctenulosis and communicable disease, especially tuberculosis. So marked was this change that as quoted by Sorsby[5] there was a reduction in phlyctenulosis in Holland of 8.7% to 1%; in Sweden from 9.5% to 1.5%; and most marked of all in Finland from 13.4% to 1.5%.

Therefore the onset of phlyctenulosis appears to require two agents. One, the prepared ground of dietary insufficiency, particularly avitaminosis C, and two, a triggering agent. This has been summarized by Rollett[9]—"a number of factors have to combine to cause this specific reaction, such as malnutrition, lack of cleanliness, vitamin deficiency, debility due to intercurrent disease and the exciting allergen, endogenous or exogenous." The fact that tuberculo-protein figures so often as the exciting allergen may be due to the fact that tuberculosis itself tends to deplete the body's reserves of vitamin C. This may be explained by the findings of Getz[10] that "it takes great quantities (3 to 4 grams daily) to establish anything that even approximates a normal blood level. It is almost impossible to saturate a tuberculosis patient with ascorbic acid when in the active phase, accompanied by fever and softening of lung tissue."

Labrador Keratopathy: The writer is in entire agreement with Freedman[2] that the etiology of this condition is due to exposure to the elements. During a recent visit to northern Newfoundland, ten patients with Labrador keratopathy were questioned. Each gave the history of sustained exposure to intense cold and glare. Typical stories were "I was snow-blind on several occasions when I was young." "I was lost in a snow-storm, I was almost dead when they found me." The most recent case gave a history of having been snow-blind every year from the age of 12 to age 65. Anyone who has been trying to reach a destination through snow and sleet, with spicules of ice hitting the eyes, which had to be kept open to find the way, can understand the trauma sustained by the exposed portion of the eye.

Pterygium: The toxic rays of sun and glare seem now to be classed as the prime cause of this condition. This has led to the conclusion by Pico[11] and Barraquer[12] that the condition is almost exclusively a disease of the tropics and sub-tropics. That this is not so is shown by the figures previously given in this article. The serious effects of short-wave light on the eye have been well documented by Duke-Elder.[13,14] A clinical study of this subject was carried out almost a hundred years ago by Gardner[15] on the snow-covered plains of the central United States. The condition of 'fishermen's lip' or actinic cheilitis, which is well known in the tropics (Marshall[16] and Nicolau[17]) is also common in Newfoundland. It has been considerably reduced since fishermen in many areas have learned to use lipstick. The validity of the idea that light rays produce the initial corneal lesion which sets the stage for pterygium formation, is borne out by the fact that all pterygium cases questioned in the recent survey had not worn sunglasses. Most of these were fishermen or woodsmen. Most of those in the former occupation are exposed to sunlight not only directly, but also by reflection from the surface either of the water or ice as in seal hunting. The high incidence of pterygium in Newfoundland fishermen is probably due to four factors:

1. The nature of employment makes the use of sunglasses difficult, as they frequently fall off and become coated with spray.
2. Refractive errors, some of which are high. To compensate for these defects, the eyelids are frequently partially shut, wrinkling the conjunctiva into horizontal folds.
3. The effect of sunlight as previously discussed, and diminished tear film as claimed by Barraquer.[12]
4. Some of the pterygia are, in fact, pseudo-pterygia, being invasions of pre-existing Labrador keratopathy by the conjunctiva.

TREATMENT

1. Prophylaxis is the keynote. This should take the form of education—encouraging the use of protective eye covering. The ivory slits which the Eskimo used to use are probably more effective against driven snow and sleet than sunglasses. They probably are just as helpful against glare during the day.

2. Steroids are useful locally in resolving the phlycten. They should be used with caution because they do not contribute to the removal of the basic vitamin deficiency and they can be dangerous in the presence of secondary infection. Large doses of vitamin C should be given orally, not only to those having

phlyctenulosis, but also those suffering from tuberculosis or other debilitating diseases.

3. Surgery is necessary when the corneal opacity in Labrador keratopathy is dense enough to reduce vision to 20/200 or less. Lamellar keratoplasty can be performed, but if no donor material is available a rotation graft can be carried out. The cornea under the upper lid in this condition is perfectly transparent and this can be used over the pupil while the opaque part of the cornea can be rotated under the upper lid. This procedure was carried out on one case in St. Anthony.

Pterygia should be surgically removed if they are active or have grown over the limbus by 2 mm. The surgical techniques are legion. All have a high recurrence rate unless the basic principle introduced by McGavic[18] is used. This consists of leaving a bare area of sclera. If the conjunctiva is sutured with 6-0 gut 3–4 mm from the limbus no irradiation with Strontium 90 has been found necessary. If the pupil has been so far encroached upon by the pterygium as to impair vision seriously, lamellar keratoplasty or rotation graft can be considered.

SUMMARY

A survey of conditions affecting the cornea in Canada's northland has been made. Congenital conditions are no more common than in other areas. The high incidence of phlyctenulosis in the Arctic is noted and its etiology is discussed. The role of vitamin C deficiency is explored.

Pterygium was found in 33% of males over 40 in a random study in northern Newfoundland. Most were fishermen. The effect of ultra-violet light in producing this lesion is discussed.

Labrador keratopathy is caused by chronic exposure to the elements of snow, sleet and glare over a period of years.

Treatment is discussed.

Acknowledgement

My thanks are due to Miss J. Hull, S.R.N., Co-ordinator of eye services of the International Grenfell Mission who compiled statistics in Newfoundland.

REFERENCES

1. Speakman, J. S. and Crawford, J. S.: Congenital opacities of the cornea. *Brit. J. Ophthal.*, 50:68, 1966.
2. Freedman, A.: Labrador keratopathy. *Arch. Ophthal. (Chicago)*, 74:198, 1965.
3. Reed, H. and Hildes, J. A.: Corneal scarring in Canadian Eskimos. *Canad. Med. Ass. J.*, 81:364, 1959.
4. Farson, C.: Phlyctenular keratoconjunctivitis at Point Barrow, Alaska. *Amer. J. Ophthal.*, 51:585, 1961.
5. Sorsby, A.: The aetiology of phlyctenular ophthalmia. *Brit. J. Ophthal.*, 26:159, 1942.
6. Stein, H. and Freiman, I.: Phlyctenular conjunctivitis in African children. *Arch. Dis. Child.*, 33:292, 1958.
7. Duke-Elder, W. S.: *Textbook of Ophthalmology. Vol. 2*. Published by H. Kimpton, London, 1938, p. 1696.
8. Holst, A. and Frolich, T. L.: Experimental studies relating to "Ship Beri-Beri" and scurvy. *J. Hyg.*, 7:634, 1907.
9. Rollet, D. M.: Allergy and its manifestations in the eyes of children. *J. of Asthma Res.*, 4:31, 1966.
10. Getz, H. R.: Problems in feeding tuberculous patients. *J. Amer. Diet. Ass.*, 30:17, 1954.
11. Pico, G.: *The Cornea World Congress*. Edited by King, J. H. and McTigue, J. W. Published by Butterworth, 1965, p. 208.
12. Barraquer, J. L.: La discontinuité localisée du film précornéen. *Ophthalmologica (Basel)*, 150:115, 1965.
13. Duke-Elder, W. S. and Duke-Elder, P. M.: A histological study on the action of short-waved light upon the eye, with a note on "inclusion bodies." *Brit. J. Ophthal.*, 13:1, 1929.
14. Duke-Elder, W. S.: The pathological action of light upon the eye. *Lancet*, 1:1137, 1926.

15. Gardner, W. H.: Account of a severe ophthalmia caused by exposure to the intense light reflected from a dazzling surface of snow. *Amer. J. Med. Sci.*, 61:334, 1871.

16. Marshall, J.: *Diseases of the Skin.* Published by E. & S. Livingstone, 1960, p. 800.

17. Nicolau, S. G. and Bulus, L.: Chronic actinic cheilitis and cancer of the lower lip. *Brit. J. Derm.*, 76:283, 1964.

18. McGavic, J. S.: Surgical treatment of recurrent pterygium. *Arch. Ophthal. (Chicago)*, 42:726, 1949.

19. Dickie, A. W.: Recurrent phlyctenular keratoconjunctivitis treated by desensitization to tuberculoprotein. *Brit. Med. J.*, Aug. 6, 1962, p. 306.

Notes

Chapter 1

1 A "tickle" in Newfoundland is a narrow strip of water between two land masses that is last to freeze up in the winter and first to break up in the spring.

2 Dr. Gordon W. Thomas, joined the Grenfell Mission in 1946 and took over the administration from Dr. Curtis, Dr. Grenfell's successor, in 1959. As the Canadian Medicare system started to pay health and hospital expenses, the dependence on external sources of funding was reduced. The final handing over of most of the International Grenfell Association (I.G.A.) assets to the newly formed Grenfell Regional Health Services Board took place early April 1981 in St. John's. Dr. and Mrs. Thomas moved to start a new life in Mabou, Nova Scotia. He has recorded the thirty-three years he spent with the Mission in his book: *From Sled to Satellite: My Years with the Grenfell Mission*, foreword by W. Anthony Paddon (Toronto: Irwin, 1987).

3 For further details of my early life in China and background, see my self-published book, *The Seed Must Grow*, 1982, ISBN 0-96-93705-0-4.

4 Dr. Walter O. Spitzer later became Professor and Chairman of the Department of Epidemiology and Biostatistics, McGill University, Senior Physician, Department of Medicine, and Director of Clinical Epidemiology, Montreal General Hospital: Professor and Associate Director, McGill Cancer Centre. Dr. Mary L. Spitzer is an Ophthalmic Surgeon at McMaster University in Hamilton, Ontario.

5 Dr. John Gray now practises internal medicine in Halifax, with special interest in geriatrics.

6 Roddickton is a community which was developed by Wilfred Grenfell as part of his plan to provide lumbering, so that those depending on fishing only, could have an extra income during the lean winter months (see Chapter 4). Sir Thomas Roddick was a native Newfoundlander who distinguished himself in medicine and became a Professor at McGill University in Montreal. During one of the periods when the ship *Strathcona* was laid up, he loaned Grenfell a "jolly-boat" to help him reach his patients in isolated coves. See W. T. Grenfell, *A Labrador*

Doctor: The Autobiography of Sir Wilfred Thomason Grenfell (London: Hodder & Stoughton, 1948) 112–13. The community was named in his honour.

Chapter 2

1 Frobisher Bay is now called "Iqaluit" ("good place for fishing"). There is some talk that the Northwest Territories may eventually divide into Eastern and Western Arctic. In light of this, and with the predominance of the Inuit in the East, some names are changing.

2 It seems that the Southern media regard the term "Eskimo" as derogatory; however, in the native language, it simply means "eater of raw meat." They almost invariably prefer to use the term "Inuit" when referring to this northern people. Like so many decisions about the North, the locals have never been consulted. They do not resent the term "Inuit," as to them it just means "survivor." By eating uncooked fish and meat these people were able to maintain a proper amount of vitamin C in their diet and hence avoided the scurvy that threatened the lives of many explorers. For further discussion see the letter to *ARCTIC: Journal of the Arctic Institute of North America*, Vol. 40, No. 4, p. 365, by the Right Reverend John R. Sperry, Bishop of the Arctic, noted linguist with thirty-seven years in the North. In the present book, the name "Inuit" is used in accordance with recent fashion.

3 The DEW (Distant Early Warning) line, a joint program of the Canadian and American governments, consists of twenty-two radar and listening posts across Alaska and the Northwest Territories. It is 5000 miles in length (3694 miles in Canada) with its eastern anchor in Broughton Island.

4 J. G. Gillan, "Canada's Northland is Challenging You," *Among the Deep Sea Fishers* (International Grenfell Association) 64 (July 1966): 41–45; reprinted in this volume as Appendix D.

5 See the biography of Elizabeth Cass by Renate Wilson, *Thank God & Dr. Cass* (Yellowknife, N.W.T.: Outcrop, 1989).

6 Elizabeth Cass, "Ocular Conditions Amongst the Canadian Western Arctic Eskimo," *Proceedings of the 20th International Congress of Ophthalmology*, International Congress Series 146 (1966) 1041–53.

7 Elizabeth Cass, "A Decade of Northern Ophthalmology: Symposium of Arctic Ophthalmology," *Canadian Journal of Ophthalmology*, 8 (1973): 210–17.

8 R. W. Morgan, J. Speakman, and S. E. Grimshaw, "Inuit Myopia: An Environmentally Induced 'Epidemic'?" *Canadian Medical Association Journal,* 112 (1975): 575–77.

9 "Symposium of Arctic Ophthalmology," *Canadian Journal of Ophthalmology,* 8 (1973): 183–310.

Chapter 3

1 Harold Horwood, *Newfoundland* (Toronto: Macmillan, 1969) 48, 76.

2 Frederick W. Rowe, *A History of Newfoundland and Labrador* (Toronto: Ryerson Press, 1980).

3 See Melvin M. Firestone, *Brothers and Rivals: Patrilocality in Savage Cove* (Institute of Social and Economic Research, Memorial University of Newfoundland, 1967) 22–23, and Thomas V. Philbrook, *Fisherman, Logger, Merchant, Miner: Social Change and Industrialism in Three Newfoundland Communities* (Institute of Social and Economic Research, Memorial University of Newfoundland, 1966) 13–14.

4 Frederick W. Rowe, *The Development of Education in Newfoundland.* (Toronto: Ryerson Press, 1964) 185–86.

5 Joseph R. Smallwood, *I Chose Canada* (Toronto: Macmillan, 1973) 194.

6 Smallwood 384.

7 Joseph R. Smallwood, *To You with Affection from Joey* (St. John's, Newfoundland: Publication Division for the Action for Joey Committees, 1969).

8 Smallwood, *I Chose Canada* 359–66.

9 Wilfred Thomason Grenfell, *A Labrador Doctor: The Autobiography of Sir Wilfred Thomason Grenfell* (London: Hodder & Stoughton, 1948) 109.

10 The Grenfell Mission could not have survived, particularly in the early days without the help of volunteers. One of the earliest of these "workers without pay" was Dr. Joseph Andrews of California, who first travelled with Dr. Wilfred Grenfell to be the first ophthalmologist to service the people of the northern peninsula and Labrador. He returned for eighteen years without pay. This must have been a formidable trip by rail and ship in those days. His picture now hangs in the Rotunda of the Charles Curtis Memorial Hospital in St. Anthony.

11 A. Freedman, "Labrador Keratopathy," *Archives of Ophthalmology (Chicago)* 74 (1965): 198.

12 Dr. W. A. (Tony) Paddon was born in Labrador at Indian Harbour where his father was in charge. After graduation, and war service he returned to Labrador, taking over the northern division of the medical service until his retirement. He was awarded the Order of Canada in 1978 and served a term as Lt.-Governor of his native province. His book, *Labrador Doctor*, was published by James Lorimer & Company in 1989.

13 G. Pico, *The Cornea World Congress*, ed. J. H. King and J. W. McTigue (London: Butterworth, 1965) 208.

14 S. G. Nicolau and L. Bulus, "Chronic actinic cheilitis and cancer of the lower lip," *British Journal of Dermatology* 76 (1964): 283.

15 W. A. Paddon, "Life in Labrador with my Famous Father," *The Book of Newfoundland, Vol. V*, ed. J. R. Smallwood (St. John's: Newfoundland Book Publishers [1967] Ltd., 1967) 489–94.

16 J. G. Gillan, R. J. Purvis, and G. W. Thomas, "Optic Atrophy Eight Years After Tuberculous Meningitis," *British Medical Journal* 4 (October 1970): 156–57.

Chapter 4

1 Helge Instad, "The Norse Discovery of Newfoundland," *The Book of Newfoundland, Vol. III*, 218–24.

2 The description of the Viking landing may seem rather imaginative, but even if we do not know exactly what happened nearly 1000 years ago, we do know from the records summarized by Helge Ingstad that Snorri was the son of Karlsefni and Gudrid, and that he was born in Vinland. Sagas differ as to whether he was three years or one year old when he left. See Ingstad's *The Norse Discovery of America, Vol. 2* (Oslo: Norwegian University Press, 1985) 129. See also Frank Ruski's article in the magazine *North*, March/April 1971. The ring-headed pin and the soapstone spindle wheel were artifacts found.

3 Dr. Gordon J. Johnson is now Professor of Preventive Ophthalmology at the Institute of Ophthalmology, University of London, and Honorary Consultant Ophtalmology at Moorfields Eye Hospital, London, England.

4 Mr. Michael Colford was formerly Director of Services, Canadian National Institute for the Blind, Newfoundland Central Region, centred in Grand Falls.

5 G. J. Johnson, J. G. Gillan, and W. G. Pearce, "Ocular Albinism in Newfoundland," *Canadian Journal of Ophthalmology*, 6 (1971): 237–48.

6 Dr. W. G. Pearce is now Professor of Ophthalmology, University of Alberta, Edmonton. *See* W. G. Pearce, G. J. Johnson, and J. G. Gillan, "Case Report: Nystagmus in a Female Carrier of Ocular Albinism," *Journal of Medical Genetics*, 9 (March 1972) 126–29. See also W. G. Pearce, R. Sanger, and R. R. Race "Ocular Albinism and Xg," *Lancet*, 1 (1968): 1282, and W. G. Pearce, J. G. Gillan, and L. Brosseau, "Bardet-Biedl Syndrome and Retinitis Punctata Albescens in an Isolated Northern Canadian Community," *Canadian Journal of Ophthalmology*, 19 (1984): 115–18.
7 S. B. Fainstein and M. R. Warren, "Community Kindergarten Vision Screening," *Canadian Journal of Ophthalmology*, 9 (1974): 425–28.
8 Ellis Shenken, "Mobile Eye Care in Newfoundland, Canada," *The Sight-Saving Review*, Winter 1971–72: 191–200.
9 J. G. Gillan, "Preventive Eye Surveys in Newfoundland and Labrador," The Canadian Ophthalmological Society Meeting, Calgary, Alberta, June 1977. See Appendices A, B, and C in this volume.
10 L. D. Wickwire, "When Kosigin Dropped In," "*Moby Joe.*" Booklet commemorating the official opening of the New Machine Room, Price (Nfld.) Pulp & Paper Limited, May 15, 1968. (First published in *The Atlantic Advocate*, August 1967.)

Chapter 5

1 H. A. Rose and T. W. D. Grant, "The Use of a Travelling Ophthalmic Technologist in a Remote, Sparsely Populated Region," *Canadian Journal of Ophthalmology*, 10 (1975): 201–04.
2 NWT Department of Social Development, Health Care Plan. *Central and Eastern Arctic Health Services Study (CEAHS)* (Yellowknife, 1977), 66.

Chapter 6

1 Joshua 14. 10–12.
2 Several of her legends appeared in *The Beaver*, a quarterly magazine published by the Hudson's Bay Company, e.g., "The Flood, Indian Legend," *The Beaver*, Spring 1960: 58; "Ojibwa Tales," *The Beaver*, Winter 1963: 58; "Cree Story of Ey-Ash-Chis," *The Beaver*, Summer 1964: 50–52. The Commissioner had authority to grant awards in two categories: conspicuous bravery, or great social service. The awards

were of two kinds: letters of commendation, or a framed citation and medal. The award given to Elizabeth Cass was of this latter variety.

3 Elizabeth Cass, *Spanish Cooking* (London: Andre Deutsch, 1957).

4 Ernie Lyall, *An Arctic Man, Sixty-five Years in Canada's North* (Edmonton, Alberta: Hurtig, 1979).

5 Farley Mowat, *The Snow Walker* (Toronto: McClelland and Stewart, 1975).

6 The story of which Ernie Lyall was critical is in the last chapter of Mowat's book, "Dark Odyssey of Soosie." Soosie was an unusually tall Inuit woman, who had gone to live on a remote Arctic Island (a result of the Hudson's Bay Company and the federal government wanting to populate the more remote areas) and who had become violently mad. Because she threatened to kill others and even to destroy the small isolated community, the rest of the group used their own method of justice and killed her. There was no policing of the area by authorities. But the two individuals involved in the actual killing were tried by "white man's law," to the shame of the Departments of Justice and Northern Affairs. If the bureaucrats in Ottawa who made the decision had ever spent a winter in the Arctic, the charges would probably never have been laid. Although the two were never to serve a jail sentence, they were broken men. Theirs was a survival decision. The Inuit had always used communal law resolutions.

7 Peter H. Bryce, *The Story of a National Crime; an Appeal for Justice to the Indians of Canada* (Ottawa: James Hope & Sons, Ltd., 1922).

8 *The Canadian Indian, Yukon and Northwest Territories.* Government of Canada, IAND Publ. No. QS-1615-000-BB-A1.

9 Ray Price, *Yellowknife* (Toronto: Peter Martin Associates Ltd., 1968) 15–18.

10 Dene Nation. *Denendeh: A Dene Celebration* (Yellowknife: The Dene Nation, P.O. Box 2338, Yellowknife, Denendeh, N.W.T. X0E 1H0) 17, and R. Fumoleau, *As Long as This Land Shall Last* (Toronto: McClelland and Stewart, 1973?) 264–68.

11 Bernie S. Siegel, *Love, Medicine and Miracles* (New York: Harper & Row, 1986) 70.

12 Elizabeth Cass, "Ocular Conditions Amongst the Canadian Western Arctic Eskimo," *Proceedings of the 20th International Congress of Ophthalmology,* International Congress Series 146 (1966) 1041–53.

13 I discussed his findings in my paper, "Reiter's Disease Among Indians in Great Slave Lake Area," *Circumpolar Health 81; Proceedings of 5th International Symposium on Circumpolar Health, Copenhagen, 9–13 August*

1981, eds. Bent Harvald and J. P. Hart Hansen (Nordic Council for Arctic Medical Research Report Series 33) 454–55.

14 Results have not been published except where I reported them in my paper (see previous note).

15 See especially: Yuri P. Nikitin, "Some Health Problems of Man in the Soviet Far North," *Circumpolar Health 84; Proceedings of the Sixth International Symposium on Circumpolar Health,* ed. Robert Fortuine (Seattle and London: University of Washington Press, 1985) 8–10, and Otto Schaefer, "Medical Research in Remote Areas and Isolated Populations: Needs, Benefits and Limitations," *Circumpolar Health 84,* 11–16.

16 Registered trademark of SmithKline Diagnostics.

17 These papers are: "Laboratory Services in the Western Arctic and Sub-Arctic (N.W.T.)," *Circumpolar Health 81,* 125–26; "3/4 of a Loaf is Better than None," Canadian Public Health Association Conference, Yellowknife, N.W.T., 1982; and "Half a Loaf is Better than None or Mini-bacteriology for Minifacilities," *Circumpolar Health 84; Proceedings of the Sixth International Symposium on Circumpolar Health,* ed. Robert Fortuine (Seattle and London: University of Washington Press, 1985) 388–89.

Index

Equipment problems, 69–71
Eskimo. *See* Inuit

Fainstein, Dr. S.B., 74
Faye, Dr. Eleanor, 1
Fisherman's lip, 54, 147
Forgie, Col. Robert, 108, 109, 111
Fort Providence, N.W.T., 90, 91, 94
Fox Creek, Alberta, 88, 89
Fraser, Ross, 41, 42
Freedman, Dr., 51, 52
Frobisher Bay, 15, 18–19, 21, 152 n.1
    hospital in, 19, 20, 24

Gander, Newfoundland, 63–64
Genetic aspects of eye defects, 54–55,
    71–74, 76–77, 119–20
Genge, Abram, 34
Glaucoma, 77
Grand Falls, Newfoundland, 62, 63
Grant, Desmond, 85
Gray, Dr. John, 5, 41, 44
Greenfield, Miss, 6, 11, 12
Grenfell, Sir Wilfred, 35–39, 47, 48, 50
    becomes doctor on mission ship, 36
    fund-raising, 38–39
    impressed by Moody, 35
    lectures, 5, 35, 36, 39
    work in education, 37
Griffiths, Mrs. Beatrice Fox, 55
Guy, John, 32

Habgood, Dr. Mary, 17, 28
Hamilton Falls. *See* Churchill Falls
    Project
Harris, Dr. Gordon, 109
Heredity and visual disorders, 26,
    54–55, 71–74, 76–77, 119–20, 141
HLA B27, 119–20
Horwood, Harold, 32
Hospitals
    Bethesda Hospital, Toronto, 3, 79
    Central Newfoundland Hospital,
        Grand Falls, 63
    Charles Curtis Memorial Hospital,
        St. Anthony, 41, 51
    Frobisher Bay, 19, 20, 24
    North York Branson Hospital,
        Toronto, 3

Northwestern General Hospital,
    Toronto, 3
Harry L. Paddon Memorial Hospi-
    tal, North West River, 51
James Paton Memorial Hospital,
    Gander, 63
Queensway Hospital, Toronto, 3
St. Anthony, 6, 14
Stanton Yellowknife Hospital,
    Yellowknife, 81, 82, 85
H.H. Williams Hospital, Hay River,
    N.W.T., 82
Hull, Nurse Jo, 10, 11, 51, 55–56,
    76–77

Igoe, Dr. Michael, 119, 120
Illiteracy as a root cause of disease, 47
Indians, 84
    eye diseases among, 118–22
    tuberculosis among, 112, 113–14
Infant mortality in the North, 37
Influenza, 114
Ingstad, Anne Stine, 65–66
Instad, Helge, 65–66
International Grenfell Association, 37,
    39, 40
International Society of Geographic
    Ophthalmology, 101, 102
Inuit
    eye problems among, 19–20, 23–24,
        25–27, 28, 112, 141–42, 143–46
    names, 106
    note on terminology, 152 n.2
    use of stenopaeic spectacles, 52, 53,
        147
ISOCULTS, 123

Johnson, Dr. Gordon J., 51, 72–73,
    154 n.3
Joint Commission of Allied Health
    Professionals in Ophthalmology
    (JCAHPO), 108, 110

Kosygin, Aleksei N., 77, 78–79
Kukreja, Dr. R., 97, 102, 108

Labrador coast (map), 7
Labrador keratopathy, 51–53, 142–43,
    146, 148